OWN the ABG

Second Edition

Associate Professor Luke D. Lawton

BAppSc (Biochemistry), MBBS (Hons) MPH (Aeromedical Retrieval)
FACEM GAICD
Staff Specialist Emergency Medicine, The Townsville Hospital
Associate Professor, College of Medicine and Dentistry
James Cook University

Dr Corinne A. Ryan

BAppSc (Biochemistry) MBBS (Hons) FRACP
Consultant Oncologist, The Townsville Hospital
Adjunct Senior Lecturer, College of Medicine and Dentistry
James Cook University

CALL the Doctors Publishing
7 St James Drive
Belgian Gardens
Townsville, Australia

National Library of Australia Cataloguing-in-Publication Data

Creator: Lawton, Luke, author.

Title: Own the ABG / Luke Lawton, Corinne Ryan

ISBN: 978-0-9924245-5-8

Notes: Includes bibliographical references.

Subjects: Blood gases - Analysis.
Clinical Biochemistry
Emergency medicine.

Other Creators/Contributors:
Ryan, Corinne, author.

Dewey Number: 616.07561

Contents

Foreword to the Second Edition

"Tell me and I forget. Teach me and I remember. Involve me and I learn."

Benjamin Franklin

When we first published *Own the ABG*, we hoped it might help a small group of our colleagues approach blood gas interpretation with more structure and less anxiety and therefore be successful in their fellowship examinations.

What we did not anticipate was how often we would be stopped in corridors at conferences, hotels, and even airports, by clinicians who have told us that the book had helped them through a difficult exam and clarified a topic that had long felt impenetrable.

Those conversations have been the most rewarding and unexpected part of this project.

Over time, however, it became clear that the original edition contained small errors and inconsistencies. None were fundamental, but some were frustrating. We were aware of them, yet the pace of clinical work and other commitments meant that revision was delayed longer than it should have been.

This second edition represents a thorough revision. The text has been carefully reviewed, calculations rechecked, explanations refined, and additional questions incorporated. The structure remains deliberately simple and exam focused. The aim has not changed: we want to provide a reproducible method for interpreting arterial blood gases under pressure.

In an era increasingly shaped by artificial intelligence, electronic medical records, and automated reporting, the ability to quickly parse and understand what a blood gas reveals about a patient's clinical state remains essential. Technology can support decision-making, but it cannot replace sound clinical judgement. Too often, when things go wrong, it is because a fundamental clinical clue has been overlooked, and often such a clue rests in a blood gas result.

Our belief remains that clarity comes from repetition, worked examples, and a disciplined approach. If this edition helps you walk into an exam with greater confidence, or (more importantly!) interpret a blood gas calmly at two in the morning in the resuscitation room, then it has served its purpose.

Thank you to the many readers who offered feedback, corrections, and encouragement. This edition exists because of you.

Luke Lawton & Corinne Ryan
25 February 2026

Foreword to OWN the ABG: what have we learnt?

"The important thing is not to stop questioning."
Albert Einstein

Since the publication of *Arterial Blood Gas Interpretation for the ACEM Fellowship Exam: 25 worked examples,* the world in some ways has changed. There is a brand new ACEM fellowship exam after all. That said, medical students, resident doctors, clinical nurses, registrars, general practitioners, and even some specialists continue to indicate to us that they still find interpreting arterial blood gases a difficult task. Therefore in many ways the world remains the same.

Our first book was focussed on a narrow audience, yet it seems to have been embraced by the medical community in countries all over the world. We were chuffed at the response to our first try at a book explaining how to break down blood gases and because of this we have expanded the scope of our book to make it accessible to all of our clinical colleagues.

We understand that for many clinicians the arterial blood gas remains a feared and poorly understood investigation. We believe that worked examples are a fantastic (and probably the outright best) method with which to undertake the difficult task of teaching an approach to the arterial blood gas.

Thus, we have produced OWN the ABG.

In this expanded version of our first book we are not trying to teach people how pass exams, although this book will certainly assist with doing so. We are trying to demystify the arterial blood gas, and take away the fear we know our colleagues feel when they are confronted with interpreting one.

The inspiration to write our first book on arterial blood gas analysis was the lack of any work teaching students how to prepare for an examination. The inspiration to produce this new book - effectively a second edition - has been a revelation that our teaching methods have assisted our colleagues in their practice.

With that said we have maintained the step wise exam focus of the original book. The clinical cases are still given and detailed in exam fashion. The suggested response to each provides a simple four step process to allow clinicians to break down, interpret, understand, and therefore utilise the arterial blood gas whether it be in the resuscitation room or by the bedside at 2am, in a rural hospital or the examination hall.

We have also added both extra worked examples, and a 30 question extended match question section. The extra questions will assist those preparing for exams, and provide a means for those who are trying to build understanding of the arterial blood gas to further test the new thought processes they have built.

We hope therefore that for anyone who takes the time to work through the examples in this book the reward will be both improved knowledge of the blood gas (and therefore success in whatever exam they study for), but more importantly an understanding that will persist for the entirety of a clinical career.

Luke Lawton and Corinne Ryan
1 May 2015

Foreword to Arterial Blood Gas Analysis for the ACEM Fellowship Exam: 25 worked examples. How to use this book.

"I'm not telling you it's going to be easy – I'm telling you it's going to be worth it."

Arthur T Williams

This book consists of 25 original questions in the style of the VAQ paper from the ACEM Fellowship exam. The questions are divided by complexity to allow each reader to judge their progress.

Each question has a worked answer, done to time (10 minutes), and some brief comments either concerning the subject matter or specific notes about the content or structure of the suggested answer. These questions have been written with specific regard to ACEM exam terminology, which can be found in the Examinations Handbook and is reproduced in the appendices here.

The worked answers are suggestions about how to produce an above average answer. Some candidates may have different opinions about the correct content of an answer. This is the nature of emergency medicine. Some of the ACEM questions are quite nebulous in their requests, particularly when it comes to "interpretation". However, all the questions given illustrate a reproducible structure for answering in the real exam, as well as practical application of relevant calculations. If you are beginning your exam preparation and are lost as to how to proceed with an ABG question the answers within should provide some guidance as to what is expected. If you are nearing the exam and within ten minutes can produce something approximating the answers in this book then you should be confident of performing well on the big day.

If you are not sitting the ACEM exam but are looking for guidance or practice on answering blood gas questions (perhaps as either as a medical student an MCEM candidate) this book still provides a useful and practical structure for interpreting the Arterial Blood Gas. Annotations of kPa equivalents for mmHg accompany all questions for those practicing in the British Isles.

We should stress that this book does not aim nor purport to offer clinical advice as to the treatment of patients. The references given for each particular section are not necessarily definitive but have been chosen because they illustrate the principles described and provide a useful springboard for further study.

The inspiration to write this book was the complete lack of any formal guides, worked examples or concentrated source of arterial blood gas questions when it came to preparing for the exam. Experience shows that these questions are a source of confusion and anxiety for candidates. This book is intended to illustrate a simple, reproducible method for answering well. We hope you find it useful.

Luke Lawton and Corinne Ryan
1 December 2013

How to interpret a blood gas in 4 easy steps.

"Success isn't always about 'greatness'. It's about consistency".
Dwayne "The Rock" Johnson

We reiterate that having a simple system with which to approach the arterial blood gas is the key to understanding the test. Our system of interpretation is a simple four step approach, which lends itself to the clinical setting as well as the examination hall.

In the worked examples section of this book the following format is used to answer ABG questions. It is adapted and altered as appropriate for each individual question, but the same process is followed for all. All calculations are included as the answer is worked and the interpretation progresses logically. Numeric headers are used as a guide through the answer. Specific notes on important calculations are provided in the appendices.

1. Acid base balance

- Comment on the pH: *acidaemia, alkalaemia*
- Comment on the CO_2: *hyper/hypocarbia, respiratory acidosis/alkalosis*
- Comment on the bicarbonate: *high/low, metabolic acidosis/alkalosis*
- Decide on the major disturbance. *This always is in the same direction as the pH.*
- Correct the dependent variable for the major disturbance. *If the primary disturbance is metabolic, correct the CO_2 for the HCO_3^-. If the primary disturbance is respiratory, correct the HCO_3^- for the CO_2. If both disturbances occur in the same direction, correct each for each other to demonstrate independence.*
- If there is a metabolic acidosis calculate an anion gap and delta ratio
- Give a summary statement of the above, for example: *"Isolated RAGMA, appropriate respiratory compensation". In clinical practice having a simple summary of the major acid-base*

disturbance established before the interpretation of the rest of the results is key to understanding the implications of your test.

2. Oxygenation

- Calculate the A-a gradient
- If you are writing an exam take the opportunity to make a comment. This can be standardised across answers, unless it is crucial to the acid-base disturbance (in the case of a respiratory acidosis and type I or type II respiratory failure).

3. Electrolytes and other numbers

- Check the electrolyte panel and comment on all minor abnormalities
- Don't forget:
    i. Correct Na^+ for glucose
    ii. Correct K^+ for pH
    iii. Calculate U:C ratio
    iv. Calculate osmolality and osmolar gap

4. Interpret and synthesise

- This is where the major list for the acid base disturbance comes into play. Highlight the major disturbances in context.

"Interpret" can be a pretty nebulous term. In examinations, the real key is to relate your answer back to the stem. To do this in either an exam or clinical practice, ask yourself:

What is the diagnosis/differential?

- Write the appropriate list and identify the most likely diagnosis for the acid base disturbance

What other tests do you need to sort out the differential diagnosis?

- Glucose for RAGMA if not given (possible DKA)
- CT brain in the obtunded patient

- Septic workup if sepsis is suspected
- Drug levels if the patient has taken an overdose (don't forget paracetamol!)
- Essentially ask yourself "what would I want the intern to have ordered for this patient?"

What are the implications of your findings?

- Likely prognosis
- Need for emergent management: antidotes, O_2, intubation, intensive care and other niceties

If you practice hard and prepare well all of that should take you a little under 10 minutes to write in detail. You should be able to think your way systematically through a blood gas and its implications in just a couple of minutes in the clinical setting.

Good luck!

A general approach to arterial blood gas questions in examinations.

"Simplicity is the ultimate sophistication"
Leonardo Da Vinci

From medical school to college and board exams examination candidates often become flustered at blood gas analysis questions. However ABG questions offer an excellent opportunity to score heavily if they are approached in an organised fashion. They are all quite similar, without the subjective vagaries of the "describe and interpret a picture" type questions and this lends itself to a systematic, repeatable approach. Ideally a candidate should write essentially the same answer every time, and just "plug in" the numbers from the question. Many examinees struggle with ABG questions because of a lack of understanding about the questions themselves, or by lacking the discipline to develop a comprehensive, simple, reproducible approach to the questions in their preparation.

There are two issues to think about when preparing for these questions.

Why is there an ABG question on the examination paper?

This is not rhetoric.

The primary reason ABG questions appear is because the question *illustrates a disturbance of acid-base metabolism that the examiners would like you to identify and describe*. There are subsequently two conclusions to draw:

i) There *will be* an acid base disturbance present in the question
ii) To pass, you need to describe it. Everything else is window dressing for bonus marks.

Within this context then, there are very few things you need to be able to talk about to answer the question properly:

i) metabolic acidosis
   - raised anion gap
   - normal anion gap

ii) metabolic alkalosis

iii) respiratory acidosis

iv) respiratory alkalosis

The list really *is* that small: 4 disorders. Having a reproducible and customisable differential for each is the key to answering the ABG question well. Such lists abound on the internet and are easily customisable. A list provided by one of the authors as an example can be found in appendix 5.

A second thought to consider about the ABG question pertains to ease of marking. In general there are a large number of calculations which can be performed by candidates and therefore marked objectively by examiners. This is an advantage for both. For examiners the question is standardised and easy to mark. For candidates the question is standardised and easy to milk. Performing calculations appropriately is critical to achieving a high mark on ABG questions. Common calculations are:

i) Anion gap

ii) Delta ratio

iii) A-a gradient

iv) Osmolar gap

v) Corrected CO_2/HCO_3^- values

vi) Electrolyte corrections, particularly Na^+ and K^+

vii) Urea:creatinine ratios

You should anticipate that examiners will be looking for these calculations with pen poised as they read your answer. However it is important not to get too obsessive about decimal points for the calculations. Often exams are conducted under extreme time pressure without a calculator. Some approximation is acceptable and will be evident in the worked examples which follow. Accuracy is important, precision less so. Of course, if you are allowed to use a calculator in your exam be very careful with rounding!

How do I answer to maximise my mark?

Begin by addressing the central acid/base imbalance

Put the question into context by ensuring you read the stem. This often gives you the diagnosis and simultaneously sets up your interpretation, yet most candidates ignore it except as the herald of a difficult ABG question. Two examples from real ACEM fellowship exams follow with comments:

Example 1.

"A 59 year old obese man receives 5 mg of intravenous morphine for analgesia for abdominal pain. Thirty minutes later, his GCS has fallen to 12 and investigations are performed." (VAQ 2009.2)

Straight away before even looking at the numbers candidates should note the following cues:

- *i)* *Obese – likely sleep apnoea, probably chronic CO_2 retention*
- *ii)* *IV morphine and decreased GCS causing acute hypoventilation and acute on chronic respiratory acidosis. This creates a need to correct HCO_3^- for both acute and chronic CO_2 retention.*
- *iii)* *This is an iatrogenic insult. Both reversal and quality assurance should be mentioned in the interpretation*

Unsurprisingly when worked these observations are exactly what the blood gas reveals.

Example 2.

"A 45 year old man with type 1 diabetes mellitus is brought in by ambulance with an altered conscious state" (VAQ 2010.1)

Straight away candidates can infer:

- *i)* *A diagnosis of DKA, and expect a showing RAGMA, Delta Ratio ~1, and profound hyperglycaemia*
- *ii)* *The possibility of a concurrent lactic acidosis due to shock/sepsis*

iii) *Probable hyponatraemia. Na^+ should be corrected for glucose*

iv) *The need for resuscitation and insulin infusion and the risk of cerebral oedema should all be mentioned in the interpretation.*

Again, these are all elements of the correct answer on working the question and reviewing the college's examination report.

Put on some window dressing as you work

Comment on minor issues as the question progresses. Don't leave everything to the end because doing so becomes rapidly overwhelming. If your comments on minor issues are inserted in the question as you work, you pick up the marks there and then and are free to concentrate on the major acid base disturbance in your interpretation. Examples of minor issues include:

i) Appropriate compensation for the major disorder

ii) A-a gradient

iii) Electrolytes:

- correct Na^+ (for glucose)
- correct K^+ (for pH)
- comment on the Cl^- if it's low. My standard comment is *"electrical equilibration for RAGMA"*
- calculate Urea:Creatinine ratio. Usually it suggests pre-renal failure
- calculated osmolality

Further information may be obtained in appendices 2 and 3.

Work through in a systematic and stepwise fashion that is easy for the examiners to follow.

Think for a moment: the examiners have to mark huge numbers of answers (50^+) in most exams. If your answer is illegible, written in hieroglyphics or algebra, or generally a dog's breakfast you are likely to be the victim of a negative free-floating marking bias. Speed is at a premium, but make sure that any abbreviations you use are common medical lexicon. A good place to start for what may be considered acceptable abbreviations is the abbreviation list contained in this book.

Essentially if you make it harder for the examiners they are likely to mark you accordingly. (If you need to be told to write legibly you should not be sitting an exam in the first instance!)

Show perspective.

Use adjectives. pH of 7.26 and 6.9 are both "acidaemias". One is a "mild" acidaemia, one is "life threatening". You want to be a consultant. Prove it.

Show sophistication: ***MUDPILES*** *is for* ***MEDICAL STUDENTS***

Have a sophisticated interpretation that conveys understanding, not rote learning. MUDPILES (causes of RAGMA) almost all present as a lactic acidosis. Writing "MUDPILES" as the differential for a RAGMA is as intellectual as withdrawing money from the "ATM machine".

There are only four significant causes of a RAGMA[1]:

i) Ketoacids;
    i. starvation
    ii. diabetes
    iii. profound dehydration (hyperemesis gravidarum, children)
ii) Lactic acid[2];
    i. type A: tissue hypo-perfusion (shock, anaemia, haemorrhage, SMA occlusion etc)
    ii. type B_1: liver failure, sepsis
    iii. type B_2: drugs (all the MUDPILES ones)
    iv. type B_3: inborn errors of metabolism. (*Editor's note: thankfully it's not a PICU fellowship exam…*)
iii) Uraemic renal failure; and
iv) Salicylates.

---

[1] Kraut JA and Madias NE. Serum anion gap: its uses and limitations in clinical medicine. *Clin J Am Soc Nephrol* 2007; 2:162-174

[2] Kriesberg RA. Lactate homeostasis and lactic acidosis. *Ann Intern Med* 1980; 92: 227-37

Rather than just reiterate a list, put something on your paper that shows understanding. Consultant opinions are characterised by clarity and sophistication.

Abbreviations.

A-a	Alveolar-arterial (oxygen gradient)
ABG	arterial blood gas
ACEM	Australasian College for Emergency Medicine
AF	atrial fibrillation
AG	anion gap
APO	acute pulmonary oedema
ARDS	adult respiratory distress syndrome
Ax	assessment
AXR	abdominal x-ray
BiPAP	bilevel positive airway pressure
BSL	blood sugar level
Ca	cancer
COPD	chronic obstructive pulmonary disease
CPAP	continuous positive airway pressure
CT	computed tomography (scan)
CTPA	computed tomography pulmonary angiogram
CVA	cerebrovascular accident
CVC	central venous catheter

CXR	chest x-ray
(D)Dx	(differential) diagnosis
DKA	diabetic ketoacidosis
DR	delta ratio
DVT	deep vein thrombosis
ECG	electrocardiogram
Ex	examination (physical)
FACEM	Fellow of the Australasian College for Emergency Medicine
FAST	focused abdominal sonography in trauma
FRACP	Fellow of the Royal Australian College of Physicians
GCS	Glasgow coma score
Hx	history
ICH	intracerebral haemorrhage
IPPV	invasive positive airway pressure
Ix	investigation
LRTI	lower respiratory tract infection
N	normal
NAGMA	normal (or non) anion gap metabolic acidosis
NAI	non-accidental injury

PE	pulmonary embolus
RAGMA	raised anion gap metabolic acidosis
RTA	renal tubular acidosis
SAH	subarachnoid haemorrhage
SIRS	systemic inflammatory response syndrome
VAQ	visual aid questions
VBG	venous blood gas
V/Q	ventilation perfusion ratio

Examination Reference Values.

It is important to have a set of easily remembered reference values that can be readily applied during the exam. The following have been used in the preparation of answers in this book:

pH	7.35 – 7.45	
PO_2	100 13.3	mmHg kPa
PCO_2	35 – 45 4.6 - 6	mmHg kPa
HCO_3^-	24	mmol/L
Base Excess	-3 to +3	
Lactate	<2	mmol/L
Na^+	135 - 145	mmol/L
K^+	3.5 – 4.5	mmol/L
Cl^-	100 – 115	mmol/L
Creatinine	<100	mmol/L
Urea	<7	mmol/L
Glucose	<6.5	mmol/L

THE EASY PROBLEMS

"'Excellent!' I cried. 'Elementary,' said he."
Sir Arthur Conan Doyle

PROBLEM 1.

A 6 year old boy presents with his parents with a five day history of profound watery diarrhoea. He is confused and drowsy at triage with a capillary refill time of 4 seconds. He is transferred to the resuscitation area and a venous blood gas is immediately taken.

Describe and interpret the results. (100%)

FiO_2	0.21		
pH	7.22		
PO_2	45	mmHg	(5.99 kPa)
PCO_2	18	mmHg	(2.4 kPa)
HCO_3^-	6	mmol/L	
BE	-18		
Na^+	140	mmol/L	
K^+	4.0	mmol/L	
Cl^-	120	mmol/L	
Urea	13	mmol/L	
Creatinine	125	µmol/L	
Glucose	2.6	mmol/L	
Lactate	1.5	mmol/L	

ANSWER

1. Acid Base Balance

Moderate acidaemia
Profound hypocapnoea
    Respiratory alkalosis

Critically low bicarbonate
    Metabolic acidosis
    Expect CO_2 = 8 + 1.5 x 6
    = 17
    .: appropriate compensation

    Anion Gap
    = 140 – 120 – 6 = 14
    Delta Ratio
    = (14 – 12)/(24-6)
    = 2/18
    <0.4 therefore Dx NAGMA

Therefore diagnose NAGMA with appropriate respiratory compensation

2. Oxygenation

A-a gradient incalculable: venous BG

3. Electrolytes

Normonatraemia
Normokalaemia
    Expect K^+ pH 7.22 = 5 + (2 x 0.5)
    = 6mmol/L
    Relative hypokalaemia, watch K^+ as pH corrected
Normochloraemia
Elevated renal indices
    U:C > 100 suggests pre-renal failure
Critically low glucose
    → requires urgent correction with 5ml/kg 10% dextrose

4. Interpret

6yo male, approx weight 20kg
Major disturbance is NAGMA
- Appropriate resp compensation
- Causes of NAGMA to consider in this child
  - HCO_3^- loss ***most likely diagnosis***
    - Diarrhoea
    - RTA (elevated renal indices)
  - Endocrinopathy
    - Addison's less likely given Na/K normal
  - Fistula
    - Pancreaticoduodenal
    - Uretoenteric
  - Drug overdose
    - Acetazolamide/spironolactone
    - Check parent's meds

Be aware NAI/neglect
- delayed presentation
- other causes of drowsiness (eg head injury)

Will need admission, fluid resuscitation 10-20ml/kg 0.9% NaCl as per APLS
Watch electrolytes
Seek and treat cause
If persistent diarrhoea consider stool culture

COMMENTS

A 6 year old boy presents with his parents with a five day history of profound watery diarrhoea. He is confused and drowsy at triage with a capillary refill time of 4 seconds. He is transferred to the resuscitation area and a venous blood gas is immediately taken.

Attention should be paid to the relevant indicators given in the stem of the question. In general, diarrhoea is associated with HCO_3^- loss and a resultant NAGMA[3]. There are also clear indicators that this child is shocked and unwell.

As may also be expected from the stem there is biochemical evidence of dehydration. Note has been made of this in the main body of the answer so as to be able to focus on the major issues in the interpretation phase. Likewise the critically low glucose has been noted and addressed, thus securing these marks prior to discussing the main metabolic disturbance. Such a critical issue is likely to represent pass/fail criteria in the exam and should not be omitted.

Finally, as this is a paediatric patient there are several "niceties" that should be observed and noted somewhere. A weight is essential (remembering the formula of (2 x age in years + 8)[4]. For a seriously unwell child to wait five days before presenting to hospital would be unusual, and raises the spectre of a child at risk. This should also be mentioned by strong candidates.

---

3 Perez GO, Oster JR and Rogers A. Acid-base disturbances in gastrointestinal disease. *Dig Dis Sci* 1978; 32(9): 1033-43

4 Luten R and Zartisky A. The sophistication of simplicity....optimizing emergency dosing. *Acad Emerg Med* 2008; 15(5): 461 - 5

PROBLEM 2

A 26 year old woman with type 1 diabetes is brought into the emergency room by the ambulance with a decreased level of consciousness. Her pathology is shown below.

Describe and interpret the results. (100%)

Serum ABG and biochemistry.

FiO_2	0.5		
pH	7.05		
PO_2	186	mmHg	(24.8 kPa)
PCO_2	66	mmHg	(8.79 kPa)
HCO_3^-	16	mmol/L	
BE	-8		
Sats	99%		
Na^+	132	mmol/L	
K^+	5.0	mmol/L	
Cl^-	92	mmol/L	
Urea	15	mmol/L	
Creatinine	227	µmol/L	
Glucose	50.9 mmol/L		

ANSWER

1. Acid base status

Critical acidaemia (pH 7.05)
Moderate hypercapnoea
    Respiratory Acidosis
    Expect HCO_3^- to be ~24-26 acutely for compensation

Moderately low bicarbonate and negative base excess
    Metabolic acidosis
    Expect pCO_2 = (20 + 0.8x16)
    = 32.8mmHg

    Anion Gap = 132 – (92+16)
    = 24

    Delta Ratio = (24 – 12)/(24-16)
    = 12/8 =1.5 (<2.0)
    Therefore Dx isolated RAGMA

Overall picture: combined respiratory acidosis and RAGMA

2. Oxygenation

A-a gradient for FiO_2 50%
= 375 – (1.25x 66) – 186
= 375 - ~80 – 186
= 295 – 186
= 109
Expect A-a grad for 45yo man = 45/4 + 4 ie 15mmHg

Therefore elevated A-a gradient suggesting respiratory shunt
    ARDS (SIRS/aspiration)
    Interstitial lung disease
    Other respiratory membrane disease (eg LRTI/APO)
    PE

3. Biochemistry

Normonatraemia
correct for glucose Na^+ = 132 + 45/3 = 147
mild elevation ?dehydrational
Mild hyperkalaemia
expect K^+ for ph 7.05 = 5 + (3 x 0.5) = 6.5 mmol/L
therefore relatively hypokalaemic and need to watch K^+ as resuscitated
Mild hyperchloraemia
Electrical equilibration RAGMA
Elevated renal indices
U:C ratio >50%
Likely some pre-renal failure 2ndary to decreased perfusion (dehydration/sepsis)
May also have element of intrinsic renal failure (diabetic nephropathy)

Profound hyperglycaemia
$Osmolality_c$ = (2 x 132) + 50 + 15 = 264 + 65
= 329mmol/Kg
HIGH
risk of cerebral oedema

4. Interpretation

This pt is critically ill:
Dx RAGMA + hyperglycaemia
Critical DKA
Needs ICU, insulin infusion and fluid/K replacement
Other causes RAGMA to consider here
Renal failure (present)
Increased lactate: check level
A – hypo-perfusion, secondary to hypovolaemia
B_1 – disease states (hepatic failure, sepsis)
B_2 – drugs especially metformin or other OD

Elevated A-a gradient and increased CO_2
Respiratory insufficiency
Concern RE aspiration given clinical history and decreased LOC

Check CXR
Septic screen as indicated

Decreased LOC and hyperosmolality
Concern RE cerebral oedema

A-a gradient in kPa

A-a gradient FiO_2 50%
= 50 kPa – (1.25 x 8.79) – 24.8
= 50 – 11 – 25
= 14 kPa

Elevated (>2.5 kPa).

COMMENTS

A 26 year old woman with type 1 diabetes is brought into the emergency room by the ambulance with a decreased level of consciousness. Her pathology is shown below.

Even a brief review of the stem will reveal the likely answer – diabetic ketoacidosis. Systemic working of the question reveals a RAGMA and a respiratory acidosis with a V/Q mismatch. To demonstrate the dual disturbance appropriate calculations are performed for both respiratory and metabolic compensation. The resultant inequity in CO_2 and HCO_3^- clearly reveals two independent processes.

This question is an illustration of several principles of answering examination ABG questions. Every calculation that can be performed should be, including in this case a calculated serum osmolality. The importance of serum osmolality in the generation of cerebral oedema remains controversial[5,6], but strong candidates will perform the calculation and hopefully pick up a mark for doing so. Corrections of Na^+ for glucose and K^+ for pH should likewise be performed. Other differentials for the RAGMA should also be mentioned, in particular lactate, which has been long described as a contributor to the acidosis in some cases of DKA[7]. As part of the interpretation the need to check a lactate therefore requires articulation. In the context of a raised A-a gradient a chest x-ray is indicated, and strong candidates will interpret the major findings as an indication for insulin therapy and disposition to a critical care area.

---

5 Tiwari LK, Jayashree M, Singhi S. Risk factors for cerebral edema in diabetic ketoacidosis in a developing country: role of fluid refractory shock. *Paed Crit Care Med* 2012; 13(2):e91-6

6 Hoorn EJ and Zietse R. Cerebral oedema in adult diabetic ketoacidosis: the importance of effective serum osmolality. *Netherlands J Med* 2010; 68(12):439

7 Watkins PJ, Smith JS, Fitzgerald MG and Malins JM. Lactic Acidosis in Diabetes. *BMJ* 1969; 1(5646): 744 - 747

PROBLEM 3

A 22 year old girl presents to ED complaining of chest pain, parasthesiae and dizziness. She has no medical history of note.

Her vital signs are:

HR	105	/min
BP	120/80	mmHg
RR	26	/min
Sats	100%	RA
Temp	37	^oC

An arterial blood gas is taken by your intern prior to registrar review and is shown below.

Describe and interpret the results. (100%)

FiO_2	0.21		
pH	7.49		
PO_2	107	mmHg	(14.3 kPa)
PCO_2	28	mmHg	(3.7 kPa)
HCO_3^-	22	mmol/L	
BE	+1		
O_2 Sats	100%		
Na^+	135	mmol/L	
K^+	4.6	mmol/L	
Cl^-	99	mmol/L	
Glucose	5.2	mmol/L	
Lactate	0.72	mmol/L	

ANSWER

1. Acid base status

Mild alkalaemia (pH 7.49)

Mild-moderate hypocapnoea
Respiratory alkalosis
Expect HCO_3^- for CO_2 28
Acute = 24 – (1 x 2) = 22mmHg
Chronic = 24 - (1 x 5) = 19mmHg

Mild decrease in HCO_3^-
Metabolic acidosis
Consistent with acute compensation for respiratory alkalosis

Therefore diagnose:
acute respiratory alkalosis
appropriate metabolic compensation

2. Oxygenation

Mild hyperoxaemia on RA
Secondary to hyperventilation

A-a gradient for FiO_2 21%
= 150 – (1.25 x 28) – 107
= 150 – 35 – 107
= 150 – 142
= 8

Expect A-a gradient 22yo female = 22/4 + 4 = 5.5 + 4 = 9.5
Not elevated
No V/Q mismatch exists

3. Electrolytes

Normonatraemia
Mild hyperkalaemia
Expect K^+ for pH = 5 - (1 x 0.5) = 4.5 mmol/L

K$^+$ level appropriate for pH
Trivial hypochloraemia
Normoglycaemia
Normal lactate

4. Interpret

ABG shows
- acute primary respiratory alkalosis with hyperoxaemia
- appropriate metabolic compensation
- no V/Q mismatch and normal vitals
  - serious pathology very unlikely

Major diagnosis is anxiety/panic attack
However multiple differentials possible
- PE: assess risk carefully PERC/Well's and Ix as appropriate
- Pneumothorax: CXR
- Drug effect or withdrawal state
  - Alcohol
  - MDMA
  - Cocaine
  - → clarify history and evaluate for toxidrome
- Pericarditis
  - Check ECG
- Pancreatitis
  - Check lipase

Issue of quality assurance
- Indication for ABG (invasive, painful) by junior doctor
- Investigate and educate as appropriate

A-a gradient in kPa

A-a gradient FiO_2 21%
$= 21 \text{ kPa} - (1.25 \times 3.7) - 14.3$
$= 21 - 4.6 - 14.3$
$= 2.1 \text{ kPa}$

Not Elevated (<2.5 kPa).

COMMENTS

A 22 year old girl presents to ED complaining of chest pain, paresthesiae and dizziness. She has no medical history of note.

An arterial blood gas is taken by your intern prior to registrar review and is shown below. Describe and interpret the results.

This is a slightly unusual stem. The first part suggests a very common ED presentation: that of acute anxiety. Consultant level perspective is given by showing awareness that the normal vital signs make occult pathology very unlikely in a young patient. However a number of serious differentials do exist for this presentation and should be mentioned in conjunction with the appropriate calculations being performed. This is essential in achieving a higher mark, and a key here is delineating extra tests which may be indicated, such as an ECG, chest x-ray or a lipase level.

The other issue which the stem prompts candidates to mention is one of quality assurance. Such issues occur intermittently within the exam, but the chance to comment for extra marks should never be missed. In this case performance of an arterial stab for blood gas analysis would seem to be overzealous, and this is an issue which should be followed up.

PROBLEM 4

An 87 year old man presents with severe central abdominal pain, vomiting and hypertension for 6 hours. He has a past history of paroxysmal atrial fibrillation and ischaemic heart disease.

His vital signs are:

HR	110	/min
BP	98/68	mmHg
RR	36	/min
Sats	100%	28% O_2
T	36.5	°C

Arterial blood gas analysis is shown below.

Describe and interpret the results. (100%)

FiO_2	0.28		
pH	7.20		
PO_2	98	mmHg	(13.0 kPa)
PCO_2	30	mmHg	(4.0 kPa)
HCO_3^-	14	mmol/L	
BE	-10		
O_2 Sats	99%		
Na^+	142	mmol/L	
K^+	5.5	mmol/L	
Cl^-	106	mmol/L	
Lactate	6.4	mmol/L	

ANSWER

1. Acid base status

Moderate acidaemia (pH 7.20)
Mild hypocapnoea
Dx respiratory alkalosis

Moderately low bicarbonate
Significant metabolic acidosis
expect CO_2 = 8 + 1.5 x 14
= 29 mmHg
.: appropriate respiratory compensation

Anion Gap
= 142 – 14 – 106
= 22 → RAGMA

delta ratio
= (22-12)/(24-14)
= 10/10
= 1.0 .: Dx isolated RAGMA
Fits with BE –10 for HCO_3^- 14

Therefore diagnose RAGMA and compensatory respiratory alkalosis.

2. Oxygenation

pO_2 → normoxia

A-a gradient for FiO_2 28%
= 200 – (1.25 x 30)– 98
= 200 – 37 – 98
= 200 – 135
= 65

Expect for 87yo male 87/4 + 4 = 22 + 4 = 26
.: Dx elevated A-a gradient → Dx V/Q mismatch
ARDS (SIRS/aspiration)
Interstitial lung disease
Respiratory membrane disease (eg LRTI/APO)

PE

3. Electrolytes

Normonatraemia
Mild hyperkalaemia
for pH 7.20 expect 5.0 + (2 x 0.5) = 6.0mmol/L
K^+ mildly low for pH
watch K^+ as pH corrected and correct if needed
Normochloraemia
Significant hyperlactataemia
Likely cause of RAGMA:
Type A - tissue hypoxia/shock
Note hypotension (bleeding, dehydration)
Vasculopath → possible mesenteric ischaemia
Type B_1 sepsis/underlying disease (eg liver failure)
Type B_2 drug OD
Possible drug toxicity: metformin, isoniazid, salicylates, paraldehyde, toxic alcohols etc

4. Interpret

ABG shows:
RAGMA with respiratory compensation
Hyperlactataemia (lactic acidosis)
Mild relative hypokalaemia
V/Q mismatch
Given Hx vomiting concern RE aspiration/ARDS

87yo male, vasculopath, AF
Concern RE catastrophic Dx
Ischaemic mesentery
Leaking AAA
Bowel obstruction
Perforated viscus
Severe sepsis
Guarded prognosis
Needs further evaluation
Renal indices/LFTs
Septic workup

Consult surgeons and radiology

CT – AAA, pneumatosis, free air

Bedside U/SS if available

Check for advanced health directive RE limits of care

A-a gradient in kPa

A-a gradient FiO_2 28%

= 28 kPa – (1.25 x 4) – 13

= 28 – 5 – 13

= 28 – 18

= 10

Elevated (>4.0 kPa).

COMMENTS

An 87 year old man presents with severe central abdominal pain, vomiting and hypertension for 6 hours. He has a past history of paroxysmal atrial fibrillation and ischaemic heart disease.

In this straightforward question the stem highlights a potentially catastrophic clinical situation. The patient is old, possesses several vascular risk factors and has severe abdominal pain. Candidates who cannot generate an appropriate differential list for this situation should not be sitting the exam! A severe metabolic acidosis should be expected as a complication of most of these illnesses[8] and this is indeed what the working reveals. Further investigations may be required to evaluate and these are briefly discussed.

The V/Q mismatch is dealt with "in question", highlighting the possibility of an aspiration, and again the K^+ is corrected appropriately. Perspective is shown by acknowledging the patient's age and guarded prognosis, and a statement that aggressive intervention may be unwarranted.

8 Lange H and Jackel R. Usefulness of plasma lactate concentration in the diagnosis of acute abdominal disease. *Eur J Surg* 1994; 160(6-7): 381-84

PROBLEM 5

Your retrieval team is tasked to pick up an 80 year old male with COPD and pulmonary oedema from a rural hospital because he requires non invasive ventilation. He has been aggressively treated with loop diuretics and nebulized salbutamol.

His venous blood gas on your arrival is shown below.

Describe and interpret the results. (100%)

FiO_2	0.21		
pH	7.58		
PO_2	66	mmHg	(8.8 kPa)
PCO_2	48	mmHg	(6.4 kPa)
HCO_3^-	38	mmol/L	
BE	+14		
O_2 Sats	89%		
Na^+	126	mmol/L	
K^+	2.2	mmol/L	
Cl^-	82	mmol/L	
Urea	8.7	mmol/L	
Creatinine	142	µmol/L	

ANSWER

1. Acid base status

Severe alkalaemia (pH 7.58)

Mild hypercapnoea
Respiratory acidosis

Significantly elevated bicarbonate
Metabolic alkalosis
expect CO_2 = 20 + (0.7 x 38)
= 20 + 26.6
= 46 mmHg
therefore appropriate respiratory compensation
AG/DR N/A for alkalosis

Therefore diagnose primary metabolic alkalosis with appropriate respiratory compensation

2. Oxygenation

Cannot be interpreted – venous sample

3. Electrolytes

Moderate hyponatraemia
Renal excretion secondary diuretics
Severe hypokalaemia
for pH 7.58 expect K^+ = 5.0 - (2 x 0.5) = 4.0mmol/L
.: K^+ still critically low when corrected for pH
Likely due to diuretic use
High risk arrhythmias/respiratory failure
Needs immediate correction with high dose IV K^+
Severe hypochloraemia
Renal excretion due to diuretics
Renal indices elevated
Urea: Creatinine ratio ~50
Implies element of intrinsic renal failure. May be medication induced

4. Interpret

ABG shows:

- Primary metabolic alkalosis with compensatory respiratory acidosis
- Multiple electrolyte deficiencies
- Life threatening hypokalaemia
- Renal failure

Metabolic alkalosis

- Diuretic induced (frusemide)
- Also consider
  - Endocrinopathies (Cushing's, Bartter's Sx)
  - HCl loss – vomiting

Respiratory acidosis

- Compensatory
- No acute indication for BiPAP at this stage: may worsen

Alkalaemia

- Needs diuretics ceased
- Urgent K+ replacement, telemetry

Iatrogenic illness

- Feed back to treating doctor
- Quality assurance procedures

COMMENTS

Your retrieval team is tasked to pick up an 80 year old male with COPD and pulmonary oedema from a rural hospital because he requires non invasive ventilation. He has been aggressively treated with loop diuretics and nebulized salbutamol.

This question is a little unusual in that the primary derangement discovered is actually an alkalaemia rather than the expected acidaemia. There is a respiratory acidosis, but this is *against* the primary direction of the pH change. Therefore it is compensatory, rather than primary. In this case the benefit of bi-level positive airway pressure is extremely dubious[9], as it will worsen the alkalaemia. There has clearly been a misinterpretation of the patient's pathology by the treating clinician.

The question also reveals multiple electrolyte elements, and an element of intrinsic renal failure[10]. There are many differentials which can be mentioned but again this question highlights the importance of returning to the stem when interpreting. In this case it highlights the cause of the problem: overzealous administration of a loop diuretic.

Once again exceptional candidates will take the opportunity to mention the issue of quality assurance. This is an iatrogenic pathology and as such should be fed back to the treating clinician.

---

9 Celikel T, Sungur M, Ceyhan B and Karakurt S. Comparison of noninvasive positive pressure ventilation with standard medical therapy in hypercapnic acute respiratory failure. *Chest* 1998; 114(6): 1636-42

10 Miller TR, Anderson RJ, Linas SL, Henrich QL, Berns AS, Gabow PA et al. Urinary diagnostic indices in acute renal failure: a prospective study. *Ann Intern Med* 1978; 89(1):47-50

PROBLEM 6

A 28 year old man presents with lethargy and dizziness. He has no medical history of note, and is a regular attendee of the local gym. He reports trying to lose weight over the last month, but denies any other symptoms.

His arterial blood gas is shown below.

Describe and interpret the results. (100%)

FiO_2	0.21		
pH	7.49		
PO_2	98	mmHg	(13.0 kPa)
PCO_2	44	mmHg	(5.9 kPa)
HCO_3^-	34	mmol/L	
BE	+10		
O_2 Sats	99%		
Na^+	132	mmol/L	
K^+	1.8	mmol/L	
Cl^-	86	mmol/L	
Urea	3.7	mmol/L	
Creatinine	62	µmol/L	

ANSWER

1. Acid base status

Mild alkalaemia (pH 7.49)

Normocapnoea

Significantly elevated bicarbonate

Metabolic alkalosis

expect CO_2 = 20 + (0.7 x 34)
= 20 + 24
= 44 mmHg

therefore CO_2 is appropriate respiratory compensation

AG/DR N/A for alkalosis

Therefore diagnose primary metabolic alkalosis with appropriate respiratory compensation

2. Oxygenation

Normoxic on RA

A-a gradient for FiO_2 21%
= 150 – (1.25 x 44) – 98
= 150 – 55 – 98
= 150 – 153
= -3

Not elevated. No V/Q mismatch.

3. Electrolytes

Mild hyponatraemia

Life threatening hypokalaemia

for pH 7.49 expect K^+ = 5.0 - (1 x 0.5) = 4.5mmol/L

.: K^+ critically low when corrected for pH

High risk arrhythmias/respiratory failure

Needs immediate correction with high dose IV K^+

Moderate - Severe hypochloraemia

Renal excretion

Renal indices normal

No obvious renal failure

4. Interpret

ABG shows:

Primary metabolic alkalosis with appropriate respiratory compensation

Life threatening hypokalaemia

Hypochloraemia

Metabolic alkalosis

Given Hx presented must consider iatrogenic

Laxative abuse

Diuretic abuse

→ needs clarification with patient

→ check other electrolytes, UA and chemistry

Other DDx include

Endocrinopathies (Cushing's, Bartter's Sx)

HCl loss – vomiting/anorexia nervosa

A-a gradient in kPa

A-a gradient FiO_2 21%

= 21 kPa – (1.25 x 5.9) – 13.0

= 21 – 7.37 – 13.0

= 0.6 kPa

Not Elevated (<2.5 kPa).

COMMENTS

A 28 year old man presents with lethargy and dizziness. He has no medical history of note, and is a regular attendee of the local gym. He reports trying to lose weight over the last month, but denies any other symptoms.

Yet again the importance of the stem cannot be overstated in answering the ABG question. We are presented with a young patient with no medical history of note, which vastly decreases the pre-test probability of serious pathology. This makes the diagnosis of iatrogenic illness much more likely. This presentation has been included in this text as a situation many examinees may not have previously encountered.

The combination of metabolic alkalosis and hypokalaemia in a healthy patient with no pathology can represent either laxative abuse[11] or diuretic abuse[12].

The critically low K^+ is dealt with during the working of the question. It is central to the answer, probably pass/fail criteria, and therefore must be mentioned. Because it is mentioned in our standard working procedure it therefore will not be missed while an interpretation of the acid-base disorder is synthesized.

The A-a gradient comes out as negative in this answer. Although this should technically be a physiologic impossibility[13] there are several possible causes to consider including recent use of supplemental oxygen, mathematical or rounding error or measurement error in the sample. It is also worth noting that there are a significant number of inherent assumptions in the calculation of an A-a gradient, and that the application of a simple equation to a complex biological system is not perfect. Overall in the event of calculating a negative gradient under

---

11 Oster JR, Masterson BJ and Rogers AI. Laxative abuse syndrome. *Am J Gastroenterol* 1980; 74(5): 451-58

12 Papademetrious V. Diuretics, hypokalemia and cardiac arrhythmia: a 20-year controversy. *J Clin Hypertens* 2006; 8(2): 86 – 92

13 Kanber GJ, King FW, Eschar YR and Sharp JT. The alveolar-arterial oxygen gradient in young and elderly men during air and oxygen breathing. *Am Rev Respir Dis* 1968; 97:376-81

exam conditions candidates would be advised to check their mathematics, and if no error is found conclude that no V/Q mismatch exists.

PROBLEM 7

An 80 year old man attends your emergency department with a humeral head fracture. He is given intravenous morphine for pain. Thirty minutes later he is noted to be drowsy and unresponsive.

His vital signs are:

HR	60	/min
BP	150/75	mmHg
RR	6	/min
Sats	90%	RA
T	36.8	°C
GCS	7	

Arterial blood gas analysis is performed and the results are shown below.

Describe and interpret them. (100%)

FiO_2	0.21		
pH	7.20		
PO_2	66	mmHg	(8.8 kPa)
PCO_2	78	mmHg	(10.4 kPa)
HCO_3^-	28	mmol/L	
BE	+2		
O_2 Sats	90%		
Na^+	136	mmol/L	
K^+	5.8	mmol/L	
Cl^-	100	mmol/L	
Glucose	6.5	mmol/L	

ANSWER

1. Acid base status

Moderate acidaemia (pH 7.20)

Significant hypercapnoea
  Respiratory acidosis
  Expect HCO_3^- for CO_2 78
    Acute = 24 + 4 = 28mmHg
    Chronic = 24 + 16 = 40mmHg

Mild-moderate increase in HCO_3^-
  Metabolic alkalosis
  Appropriate acute compensation for CO_2 78mmHg

Therefore diagnose acute respiratory acidosis with appropriate metabolic compensation.

2. Oxygenation

Critical hypoxia on room air
  Administer supplemental O_2
  Type II respiratory failure

A-a gradient FiO_2 21%
$$= 150 – (1.25 \times 78) – 66$$
$$= 150 – 100 – 66$$
$$= 150 – 166$$
$$= -16$$

Not elevated
No V/Q mismatch
  Hypoxia likely due to pure hypoventilation

3. Electrolytes

Normonatraemia
  Not cause of obtundation

Mild hyperkalaemia

Expect K^+ for pH = 5 + (2 x 0.5) = 6.0 mmol/L

K^+ level appropriate for pH

Normochloraemia

Mild hyperglycaemia

Not cause for decreased GCS

4. Interpret

ABG shows acute respiratory acidosis with appropriate metabolic compensation.

Given clinical history strongly suggests opiate induced hypoventilation.

- Also consider
  - Intracerebral insult
    - CVA
    - ICH/SAH
    - Undiagnosed head injury (ExDH, SDH)
  - Secondary cause of low GCS
    - Sepsis

Vital signs show obtundation and hypoventilation

- Trial of reversal : naloxone
- If no success may need airway support
- No evidence of haemodynamic compromise as cause of low GCS

Likely iatrogenic insult

- Review case
- Quality assurance procedures
- Open disclosure to patient/family

A-a gradient in kPa

A-a gradient FiO_2 21%
= 21 kPa – (1.25 x 10.4) – 8.8
= 21 – 13 – 8.8
= <0 kPa

Not Elevated (<2.5 kPa).

COMMENTS

An 80 year old man attends your emergency department with a humeral head fracture. He is given intravenous morphine for pain. Thirty minutes later he is noted to be drowsy and unresponsive.

Once again the stem sets up a fairly obvious answer. This patient is likely to have an iatrogenic suppression of respiration due to administration of opiates. Candidates should therefore expect an acutely compensated respiratory acidosis which is what the working indeed shows. The significance of a negative A-a gradient was discussed in problem 6.

Better candidates will also recognize the possibility of other causes of a decreased GCS with the given history of trauma. Again as an iatrogenic insult it is very important to mention relevant quality assurance issues. The principle of open disclosure is a key issue in the management of medical errors and should be mentioned for high marks[14]. The examiners here create potential opportunity to score higher marks by showing consultant level perspective.

14 Iedema RA, Mallock NA, Sorensen RJ, Manias E, Tuckett AG, Williams AF et al. The national open disclosure pilot: evaluation of a policy implementation initiative. *MJA* 2008; 188(7):397-400

PROBLEM 8

An 80yo female with a history of rheumatoid arthritis presents with acute confusion. She lives alone and has not been seen for 2 days.

Her blood gas is shown below.

Describe and interpret the results. (100%)

FiO_2	0.21		
pH	7.16		
PO_2	100	mmHg	(13.3 kPa)
PCO_2	28	mmHg	(3.7 kPa)
HCO_3^-	14	mmol/L	
BE	-8		
Na^+	120	mmol/L	
K^+	7.6	mmol/L	
Cl^-	100	mmol/L	
Glucose	4.0	mmol/L	
Lactate	1.2	mmol/L	

ANSWER

1. Acid-Base Balance

Moderate acidaemia
Significant hypocapnoea
Respiratory alkalosis
Moderately low HCO_3^-
Metabolic Acidosis
Expect CO_2 = 8 + (1.5 x 14)
= 29
.: appropriate compensation
Anion Gap
= 120 – 100 – 14
= 6
.: Dx NAGMA

Delta R not calculable as AG <12 (ie N)

Therefore Dx NAGMA with appropriate respiratory compensation

2. Oxygenation

Gross normoxia

A-a gradient FiO_2 21%
= 150 – (1.25 x 28) – 100
= 150 – 35 – 100
= 115 – 100
= 15

Expect A-a for 80yo = 80/4 + 4 = 24
.: Dx N A-a gradient
No V/Q mismatch

3. Electrolytes

Significant hyponatraemia
Evaluate hydration status and medications (SSRI etc)
Needs correction 0.5mmol/L.hr

Profound hyperkalaemia

Expect K^+ pH 7.16 = 5.0 + (2.5 x 0.5)

= 6.125mmol/L

Therefore absolutely hyperkalaemic

Check ECG

Normochloraemia

NAGMA

Normoglycaemia

Not cause of confusion

Normal lactate

Less likely to be severely septic/shocked

4. Interpret

NAGMA plus hyponatraemia and hyperkalaemia

Likely adrenal insufficiency

Pt has RA – possible long term steroid use

Supplemental steroids indicated

DDx for NAGMA in this setting: needs further evaluation for:

Drugs – spironolactone, acetazolamide

Fistula – uretoenteric, pancreaticoduodenal

Renal failure – check renal indices and urine

HCO_3^- loss – diarrhoea

Panhypopituitarism

Adrenal necrosis (Waterhouse-Friedrichson syndrome) if septic

Other things to consider

Not seen 2 days

Long lie syndrome

Evaluate renal function and CK

Drowsiness/confusion

Evaluate other causes

Septic screen, CT head

A-a gradient in kPa

A-a gradient FiO_2 21%
= 21 kPa – (1.25 x 3.7) – 13.3
= 21 – 4.6 – 13.3
= 3.1 kPa

Not Elevated for age (<4.0 kPa for 80yo).

COMMENTS

An 80yo female with a history of rheumatoid arthritis presents with acute confusion. She lives alone and has not been seen for 2 days.

This stem is somewhat vague and represents a host of possibilities in this geriatric patient. It is an illustration of the need to both work through the question systematically, but also to consider the underlying possibilities and include these in the interpretation.

Systematic working of the question will reveal a NAGMA with associated hyponatraemia and hyperkalaemia, and the stem suggests the possibility of steroid use. Together this paints the picture of an acute adrenal crisis. Purists will argue that acute adrenal crisis complicated by hyperkalaemia and hyponatraemia only occurs in primary adrenal insufficiency, because the pathophysiologic process is mediated by failure of mineral corticoid secretion [15]. Although classically steroid withdrawal only results in glucocorticoid deficiency, chronic adrenal fatigue and resultant acute adrenal crisis has been reported in patients undergoing long term glucocorticoid therapy [16]. The possibility of intercurrent sepsis and Waterhouse-Friedrichson syndrome (true adrenal crisis) should also be mentioned given the clinical picture, as should the possibility of excessive spironolactone use.

15 Burke CW. Adrenocortical insufficiency. *Clin Endocrinol Metab* 14(4): 947 -76

16 Cronin CC, Callaghan N, Kearney PJ, Murnaghan DJ and Shanahan F. Addison disease in patients treated with glucocorticoid therapy. *Arch Intern Med* 1997; 157(4):456 -8.

Strong candidates will also note the differential diagnosis for a NAGMA in their answer, and mention the possibility of a "long-lie" syndrome, which could also be associated with many of the electrolyte abnormalities described in the stem[17]. Thus renal function and a creatine kinase level should be urgently requested as part of the candidates "interpretation" of this question. Finally given the acute confusional state a CT brain should be considered.

---

17 Szewczyk D, Ovadia P, Abdullah F and Rabinovici R. Pressure-induced rhabdomyolysis and acute renal failure. *J Trauma* 1998; 44(2): 384 - 8

PROBLEM 9

A 48 year old man presents complaining of nausea. He had a root canal two days ago and has consumed 26 compound paracetamol/codeine tablets in the last 24 hours for pain.

Selected investigations are shown below.

Describe and interpret the results. (100%)

FiO_2	0.21		
pH	7.02		
PO_2	109	mmHg	(14.5 kPa)
PCO_2	19	mmHg	(2.5 kPa)
HCO_3^-	8	mmol/L	
BE	- 16		
O_2 Sats		100%	
Na^+	138	mmol/L	
K^+	6.3	mmol/L	
Cl^-	103	mmol/L	
Lactate	12.6	mmol/L	
Glucose	5.4	mmol/L	
AST	6500	IU/L	
ALT	5900	IU/L	
GGT	65	IU/L	
ALP	106	IU/L	
Bilirubin	50	mmol/L	

ANSWER

1. Acid base status

Life threatening acidaemia (pH 7.02)
Critical hypocapnoea
Dx respiratory alkalosis

Severely low bicarbonate
Critical metabolic acidosis
expect CO_2 = 8 + (1.5 x 8)
= 20 mmHg
.: appropriate respiratory compensation

Anion Gap
= 138 – 8 – 103
= 27 → RAGMA

Delta Ratio
= (27-12)/(24-8)
= 15/16
= 1.0 .: Dx isolated RAGMA
Fits with BE –16 for HCO_3^- 8

Therefore diagnose RAGMA and compensatory respiratory alkalosis.

2. Oxygenation

pO_2 → mild hyperoxia

A-a gradient for FiO2 21%
= 150 – (1.25 x 19) – 109
= 150 – 25 – 109
= 150 – 136
= 14
Expect for 45yo male 45/4 + 4 = 11 + 4 = 15
.: Dx N A-a gradient
No V/Q mismatch exists

3. Electrolytes

Normonatraemia

Moderate hyperkalaemia

for pH 7.02 expect 5.0 + (4.0 x 0.5) = 7.0mmol/L

K^+ mildly low for pH

watch K^+ as pH corrected and correct if needed

Borderline hypochloraemia

Electrical equilibration for RAGMA

Normoglycaemia

Grossly deranged liver function

Hepatocellular picture

Complicated by hyperbilirubinaemia

Check conjugated fraction

Likely paracetamol induced hepatotoxicity given history

Critical hyperlactataemia

Likely cause of RAGMA:

Type A - tissue hypoxia/shock

Type B_1 sepsis/underlying disease (eg liver)

Paracetamol Hepatotoxicity

Type B_2 drug OD

Possible drug toxicity: metformin, isoniazid, salicylates etc

4. Interpret

ABG shows:

Critical Lactic acidosis plus acute hepatitis

Appropriate respiratory compensation

Mild relative hypokalaemia

needs monitoring

Probable paracetamol induced hepatotoxicity

Obtain levels as proof

Screen for other causes

Hepatitis serology

Ultrasound scan

Needs **immediate** treatment with NAC

ICU and gastroenterology consults

Guarded prognosis → may require liver transplant

A-a gradient in kPa

A-a gradient FiO_2 21%
= 21 kPa – (1.25 x 2.5) – 14.5
= 21 – 3.13 – 14.5
= 3.37 kPa

Borderline elevation (>2.5 kPa).

COMMENTS

A 48 year old man presents complaining of nausea. He had a root canal two days ago and has consumed 26 compound paracetamol/codeine tablets in the last 24 hours for pain.

Even a brief read of the stem should enlighten the examinee as to the diagnosis of paracetamol hepatotoxicity. Over-ingestion of paracetamol leads to the formation of an electrophilic toxic metabolite[18], NAPQI, which causes centrilobular hepatic necrosis[19].

The question itself is a straightforward case of RAGMA associated with lactic acidosis, and should be worked as such. The deranged liver function indicates that this patient is at risk of life threatening paracetamol poisoning, and must be treated immediately with N-Acetyl Cysteine. Mentioning this is essential, even though the data regarding delayed administration indicates poorer prognosis[20].

For completeness sake strong candidates will comment on relevant minor issues, specifically correction of the K^+, the hyperbilirubinaemia and the

18 Manyike PT, Kharasch ED, Kalhorn TF and Slattery JT. Contribution of CYP2E1 and CYP3A to acetaminophen reactive metabolite formation. *Clin Pharmacol Ther* 2000; 67(3):275-82

19 Lee WM. Drug-induced hepatotoxicity. *NEJM* 2003; 349(5):474-485

20 Smilkstein MJ, Bronstein AC, Linden C, Augenstein WL, Kulig KW and Rumack BH. Acetaminophen overdose: a 48-hour intravenous N-acetylcysteine treatment protocol. *Ann Emerg Med* 1991; 20(10):1058-63

need to measure a conjugated fraction, and the need to consider other causes of liver dysfunction. Finally, perspective is shown by obtaining relevant consults and mentioning the gravity of the prognosis.

PROBLEM 10

A 45 year old woman presents to your department complaining of 6kg weight gain and lethargy over the last 3 weeks. She is not on medication and has been previously healthy, and says she thinks she has begun menopause.

Her vital signs are:

HR	80	/min
BP	165/90	mmHg
RR	12	/min
Sats	98%	RA
T	37.1	°C

An arterial blood gas is taken and the results are shown below.

Describe and interpret them. (100%)

FiO_2	0.21		
pH	7.51		
PO_2	102	mmHg	(13.6 kPa)
PCO_2	44	mmHg	(5.9 kPa)
HCO_3^-	34	mmol/L	
BE	+10		
O_2 Sats	98%		
Na^+	152	mmol/L	
K^+	2.2	mmol/L	
Cl^-	122	mmol/L	
Glucose	11.5	mmol/L	

ANSWER

1. Acid base status

Moderate alkalaemia (pH 7.51)

Normocapnoea

Moderately elevated HCO_3^-

Metabolic alkalosis

expect CO_2 = 20 + (0.7 x 34)
= 20 + 23
= 43 mmHg

therefore CO_2 is appropriate compensation

AG/DR not applicable for metabolic alkalosis

Therefore diagnose primary metabolic alkalosis with appropriate respiratory compensation.

2. Oxygenation

Normoxic on RA

A-a gradient FiO_2 21%

= 150 – (1.25 x 44) – 102
= 150 – 55 – 102
= -7

Not elevated

Implies no V/Q mismatch

3. Electrolytes

Mild-moderate hypernatraemia

Critical hypokalaemia

Expect K^+ for pH = 5 - (1 x 0.5) = 4.5 mmol/L

Therefore grossly K^+ deficient

High risk arrhythmia

Needs urgent replacement and telemetry monitoring

Mild hyperchloraemia

Moderate hyperglycaemia

Undiagnosed diabetes

Steroid therapy
Other endocrinopathy (eg Cushing's Sx)

4. Interpret

ABG shows:
- Metabolic alkalosis with appropriate respiratory compensation
- Critical hypokalaemia
- Moderate hyperglycaemia

Causes of metabolic alkalosis
- Endocrinopathy
  - Cushing's syndrome
    - Primary
    - Secondary
    - Paraneoplastic
    - Iatrogenic (check medication Hx for steroids)
  - Hyperaldosteronism
  - Bartter's Sx
- HCl loss
  - Check if vomiting
- Drugs
  - Frusemide/other diuretics: less likely with weight gain

Overall suggests Cushing's Sx
- Correlate clinically (striae, body habitus etc)
- Endocrine consult
  - Check other electrolytes and renal Fn
  - Urine chemistry
  - Consider further Ix (cortisol levels) and imaging (MR/CT brain and abdomen) in consult
- Replace K^+
  - High dose IV either KCl or KH_2PO_4
  - Telemetry environment for same

A-a gradient in kPa

A-a gradient FiO_2 21%
= 21 kPa – (1.25 x 5.9) – 13.6
= 21 – 7.38– 13.6
= 0.02 kPa

Not Elevated (<2.5 kPa).

COMMENTS

A 45 year old woman presents to your department complaining of 6kg weight gain and lethargy over the last 3 weeks. She is not on medication, has been previously healthy, and says she thinks she has begun menopause.

The stem suggests a nonspecific constellation of symptoms which are revealed to be associated with a metabolic alkalosis after working the question. The most likely cause is an endocrinopathy, and the triad of metabolic alkalosis, hypokalaemia and hypertension may represent either an excessive glucocorticoid (Cushing's) or mineralocorticoid (Conn's) syndrome[21,22].

In this case the clinical information given in the stem and the glucose intolerance favour a diagnosis of Cushing's syndrome, but both differentials should be mentioned, as well as the need to consult endocrinology. Giving a broader differential for the diagnosis of metabolic alkalosis is likely to earn more marks.

---

21 Torpy DJ, Mullen N, Ilias I and Nieman LK. Association of hypertension and hypokalemia with Cushing's syndrome caused by ectopic ACTH secretion: a series of 58 cases. *Ann N Y Acad Sci* 2002; 970:134-44

22 Stewart PM. Mineralocorticoid hypertension. *Lancet* 1999; 353(9161):1341-7

PROBLEM 11

A 58 year old woman on chemotherapy for breast cancer presents to your department feeling generally unwell.

Her vital signs are:

HR	105	/min
BP	110/65	mmHg
RR	28	/min
Sats	92%	6L
T	38.6	°C

Her ABG is shown below.

Describe and interpret the results. (80%)

List further investigations you would consider. (20%)

FiO_2	0.40		
pH	7.28		
PO_2	68	mmHg	(9.0 kPa)
PCO_2	40	mmHg	(5.3 kPa)
HCO_3^-	18	mmol/L	
BE	-6		
O_2 Sats	92%		
Na^+	141	mmol/L	
K^+	4.6	mmol/L	
Cl^-	106	mmol/L	
Glucose	5.8	mmol/L	

ANSWER

1. Acid base status

Mild acidaemia (pH 7.28)
Normocapnoea

Mildly low bicarbonate
Mild metabolic acidosis
expect CO_2 = 8 + (1.5 x 18)
= 35 mmHg
.: inadequate respiratory compensation
Relative respiratory acidosis

Anion Gap
= 141 – 18 – 106
= 141 - 124
= 17 → RAGMA

delta ratio
= (17-12)/(24-18)
= 5/6
= ~1.0 .: Dx isolated RAGMA
Fits with BE –6 for HCO_3^- 18

Therefore diagnose RAGMA and compensatory respiratory alkalosis.

2. Oxygenation

pO_2 → significant hypoxia on supplemental O_2

A-a gradient FiO_2 40%
= 300 – (1.25 x 40) – 68
= 300 – 50 – 68
= 300 – 118
= 182

Expect for 58yo female 58/4 + 4 = 14 + 4 = 18
.: Dx elevated A-a gradient → Dx V/Q mismatch
Concerning for LRTI/PE given sats and Hx

ARDS (SIRS/aspiration)
Interstitial lung disease
Other respiratory membrane disease (eg APO)

3. Electrolytes

Normonatraemia
Normokalaemia
for pH 7.28 expect 5.0 + (1 x 0.5) = 5.5mmol/L
.: K^+ very mildly low for pH
watch K^+ as pH corrected
Normochloraemia
Normoglycaemia
DKA unlikely as cause of RAGMA

4. Interpret

ABG shows:
RAGMA with inadequate respiratory compensation (acidosis) and V/Q mismatch

Febrile cancer pt on chemotherapy
High risk sepsis
Needs broad spectrum empiric Abx (gentamicin + pip/taz or cefepime)

RAGMA causes to consider:
Lactate: check level
A – shock/tissue hypoxia
B_1 – sepsis, liver failure (mets)
LRTI, urosepsis, line sepsis if vascular access device
B_2 – drugs: iron, isoniazid, paraldehyde, metformin, toxic alcohols
Ketones
DKA unlikely with N BSL
Starvation
Dehydration
Renal failure
Dehydration, chemotherapy

V/Q mismatch

Febrile – concern RE LRTI. PE also more likely given Hx Ca

Therefore based on above, further Ix are:

Bedside:

ECG

Urine dip

Pathology:

FBC (WCC/Hb)

E/LFTs (renal fn, liver Fn, lipase, Ca^{++})

Lactate (sepsis)

Septic screen - Urine culture, BCs x 2 sets plus line, CXR

Drug levels if indicated

CSF m/c/s if concern RE meningitis

Imaging

CXR

CTPA if no cause for V/Q MM found

Other imaging as clinically indicated

U/SS ?DVT

CT abdomen or U/SS if abdominal focus suspected

A-a gradient in kPa

A-a gradient FiO_2 40%

= 40 kPa – (1.25 x 5.3) – 9

= 40 – 6.63 – 9

= 24.37 kPa

Grossly elevated (>2.5 kPa).

COMMENTS

A 58 year old woman <u>on chemotherapy</u> for breast cancer presents to your department feeling generally unwell.

Her vital signs are:

HR	*105*
BP	*110/65*
RR	*28*
Sats	*92% 6L*
T	*38.6°C*

Candidates will notice that the stem gives three very important pieces of information: fever and hypoxia in a patient on chemotherapy. This is a situation than mandates empiric antibiotics[23] and this should be made clear in the candidate's answer.

There are also two questions given. There is the usual "describe and interpret" prompt, but also a request for a "list" of further investigations. This should be regarded by the candidates as a request for a focused interpretation of the information given, rather than a need to generate an entirely new answer halfway through the question. In this case the clinical need will be to evaluate for a cause for the fever, and a cause for the elevated A-a gradients. Fellowship level candidates should generate an appropriate list of investigations without much difficulty.

23 Flowers CR, Seidenfeld J, Bow EJ, Karten C, Gleason C, Hawley DK et al. Antimicrobial prophylaxis and outpatient management of fever and neutropenia in adults treated for malignancy: American Society of Clinical Oncology clinical practice guideline. *J Clin Oncol* 2013; 31(6):794-810

PROBLEM 12

A 26 year old man presents with dyspnoea and weakness. His parents mention that he has a history of "kidney problems" and that he has not been compliant with his medication.

His arterial blood gas on arrival is shown below.

Describe and interpret the results. (100%)

FiO_2	0.21		
pH	7.08		
PO_2	110	mmHg	(14.7 kPa)
PCO_2	19	mmHg	(2.5 kPa)
HCO_3^-	7	mmol/L	
BE	-16		
O_2 Sats	100%		
Na^+	136	mmol/L	
K^+	1.8	mmol/L	
Cl^-	124	mmol/L	
Urea	4.7	mmol/L	
Creatinine	42	µmol/L	

ANSWER

1. Acid base status

Severe acidaemia (pH 7.08)

Profound hypocapnoea
Respiratory alkalosis

Severely low bicarbonate
Metabolic acidosis
expect CO_2 = 8 + (1.5 x 7)
= 18 mmHg
therefore appropriate respiratory compensation

Anion Gap
= 136 – 7 – 124
= 136 – 131
= 5 → NAGMA

DR n/a as AG < 12

Therefore diagnose NAGMA with appropriate respiratory compensation

2. Oxygenation

pO_2 → mildly hyperoxic on RA
probably secondary to hyperventilation due to respiratory compensation

A-a gradient FiO_2 21%
= 150 – (1.25 x 19) – 119
= 150 – 25 – 119
= 150 – 144
= 6

Expect for 26yo male 26/4 + 4 = 4.5 + 4 = 8.5
.: N A-a gradient. No V/Q mismatch

3. Electrolytes

Normonatraemia

Critical hypokalaemia

for pH 7.08 expect K^+ = 5.0 + 3 x 0.5 = 6.5mmol/L

.: K^+ life threateningly low when corrected for pH

High risk arrhythmias/respiratory failure

Needs immediate correction with high dose IV K^+

Hyperchloraemia

NAGMA

Renal indices normal

No evidence renal failure as cause for NAGMA

Interpret

ABG shows:

NAGMA with appropriate respiratory compensation

Critical hypokalaemia

Findings consistent renal tubular acidosis

Check urine pH (>5.3)

Check other electrolytes, esp Ca^{++}

pH may respond to HCO_3^- administration

Other causes of NAGMA to consider

Hypoaldosteronism

Adrenal insufficiency

Spironolactone use

Acetazolamide use

NaCl administration

Renal failure (unlikely with N indices)

Critical hypokalaemia

Needs high dose K^+ replacement IV

Telemetry/HDU involvement: high risk arrhythmia and respiratory failure

A-a gradient in kPa

A-a gradient FiO_2 21%
= 21 kPa – (1.25 x 2.5) – 14.7
= 21 – 3.13 – 14.7
= 3.17 kPa

Mild elevation (>2.5 kPa).

COMMENTS

A 26 year old man presents with dyspnoea and weakness. His parents mention that he has a history of "kidney problems" and that he has not been compliant with his medication.

Candidates reading this stem may be perplexed as to the underlying implications. A good place to start with questions like this with no underlying clue to diagnosis in the stem is with systemic working to elucidate the major abnormalities. In this question these are NAGMA and hypokalaemia. In keeping with the practice of commenting on non acid-base issues during working of the question the importance of the hypokalaemia is identified and dealt with "in question". This is the likely cause of the patient's weakness[24], and will need to be urgently corrected. This is likely to be a pass/fail criteria.

Once the NAGMA is identified the list of differentials can be revisited to find a link with the information given in the stem. In this case renal loss of HCO_3^- is a likely to be relevant and should be articulated as such.

Both proximal tubular renal tubular acidosis (with or without Fanconi syndrome) and distal renal tubular acidosis are associated with NAGMA

24 Comi G, Testa D, Corneolio F, Comola M and Canal N. Potassium depletion myopathy: a clinical and morphological study of six cases. *Muscle Nerve* 1985; 8(1):17 - 21

and hypokalaemia[25, 26], although the disturbances tend to be more severe with distal disease. Often patients with these conditions are maintained on bicarbonate therapy, presumably the medication with which this young man has not been compliant. It is very important to mention both the need to evaluate the other electrolytes, and to urgently replace the potassium in this patient as part of a sophisticated consultant level interpretation.

---

25 Sebastian A, McSherry E, and Morris RC Jr. Renal potassium wastin in renal tubular acidosis (RTA): its occurrence in types 1 and 2 RTA despite sustained correction of systemic acidosis. *J Clin Invest* 50(3): 667 – 78

26 Batle D, Moorthi KM, Schlueter W and Kurtzman N. Distal renal tubular acidosis and the potassium enigma. *Semin Nephrol* 2006; 26(6): 471-8

PROBLEM 13

A 26 year old mechanic is brought in by ambulance after an overdose of an unknown substance. On arrival his vital signs are:

HR	106	/min
BP	80/50	mmHg
RR	34	/min
sats	100%	RA
GCS	12	/min

An arterial blood gas drawn on arrival in the resuscitation area is shown below.

Describe and interpret the results. (100%)

FiO_2	0.21		
pH	7.15		
pO_2	116	mmHg	(15.4 kPa)
pCO_2	20	mmHg	(2.7 kPa)
HCO_3^-	8	mmol/L	
BE	-16		
Na^+	135	mmol/L	
K^+	6.5	mmol/L	
Cl^-	95	mmol/L	
glucose	6.2	mmol/L	
urea	8.1	mmol/L	
lactate	5.2	mmol/L	
measured osmolality	320	mosm/Kg	

ANSWER

1. Acid-Base Balance

Severe acidaemia (7.15)
Moderate hypocapnoea
respiratory alkalosis
Severely low HCO_3^- and large -ve BE
metabolic acidosis
expect CO_2 = 8 + (1.5 x 8)
= 20mmHg
.: diagnose appropriate respiratory compensation
Anion Gap
= 135 - 95 - 8
= 32
Delta ratio
= (32 - 12)/(24 - 8)
= 20/16
= 1.25
.: diagnose isolated RAGMA

Therefore Dx RAGMA with appropriate resp compensation

2. Oxygenation

Mild hyperoxaemia on room air
A-a gradient FiO2 21%
= 150 - (1.25 x 20) - 116
= 150 - 25 - 116
= 9

Expect A-a 20yo = 20/4 + 4 = 9

N A-a gradient. No V/Q mismatch exists.

3. Electrolytes

Normonatraemia
Hyperkalaemia
expect K^+ for pH 7.15 = 5 + (2.5 x 0.5)

= 5 + 1.25

= 6.25mmol/L

.: K^+ 6.5 is appropriate for pH

Mild hypochloraemia

electrical equilibration RAGMA

Normoglycaemia

not cause ALOC

Significant hyperlactataemia

type A: hypoperfusion/shock

type B_1: sepsis/liver failure. Check LFT

type B_2: drugs

Metformin, iron, toxic alcohols, isoniazid, paraldehyde, paraquat

Hyperosmolar state

risk cerebral oedema

osmolar gap $= osm_c - osm_m$

= 320 - (2 x Na + urea + glucose)

= 320 - 270 - 8 - 6

= 50 - 14 = 36 ie high

STRONGLY implies toxic alcohol ingestion

check urine for oxalate

check formic acid levels

4. Interpret

Overdose, young man, severe metabolic compromise

compensated RAGMA plus raised osm gap

suggests ethylene glycol or methanol intoxication

urgent treatment indicated

antidotes: ethanol or fomepizole. Consult toxicology

haemodialysis likely indicated: consult ICU

needs paracetamol level (co-ingestant)

psych input as required

evaluate for other causes of lactate: septic screen, GI bleed etc

A-a gradient in kPa

A-a gradient FiO_2 21%
= 21 kPa – (1.25 x 2.7) – 15.4
= 21 – 3.38 – 15.4
= 2.22 kPa

Not Elevated (<2.5 kPa)

COMMENTS

A 26 year old mechanic is brought in by ambulance after an overdose of an unknown substance.

Interestingly the stem here provides little clue as to the pathologic process examinees are expected to delineate. However a major clue may be garnered from examining the results candidates are expected to work:

measured osmolality 320 mosm/Kg

There are few reasons to provide a measured osmolality to candidates, unless the examiners expect calculation of an osmolar gap. In the setting of an overdose, this strongly implies the possibility of either methanol or ethylene glycol ingestion[27]. Candidates should expect a concurrent RAGMA with a high lactate. Systematic working of the question does indeed reveal these findings. Of note, calculating the DR reveals an answer >1.0. However this should not be interpreted as a concurrent metabolic alkalosis. Small deviations about 1 probably reflect an inherent inaccuracy in the method of calculation, and a metabolic alkalosis is unlikely unless the ratio exceeds 2.

To score highly candidates should demonstrate their understanding of the subject by reference to specific metabolites of methanol (formic acid)[28]

27 Lynd LD, Richardson KJ, Purssell RA, Abu-Laban RB, Brubacher JR, Lepik KJ et al. An evaluation of the osmole gap as a screening test for toxic alcohol poisoning. *BMC Emerg Med* 2008; 8:5

28 D'Alessandro A, Osterloh JD, Chuwers P, Quinlan PJ, Kelly TJ and Becker CE. Formate in serum and urine after controlled methanol exposure at the threshold limit value. *Environ Health Perspect* 1994; 102(2):178-81

and ethylene glycol (oxaloacetate)[29]. Relevant treatment by either inhibition of alcohol dehydrogenase inhibition[30] or haemodialysis should also be highlighted. The indications for haemodialysis are controversial, but include the presence of RAGMA, end organ damage or an osmolar gap >10[30]. Expert opinion should be sought.

Finally, good candidates, realizing that this is a potential episode of self harm should mention the need to test for co-ingestants and seek appropriate input from toxicology, intensive care and psychiatry services.

---

29 Fraser AD. Clinical toxicologic implications of ethylene glycol and glycolic acid poisoning. *Ther Drug Monit* 2002; 24(2):232-8

30 Barceloux DG, Krenzelok EP, Olson K and Watson W. American Academy of Clinical Toxicology Practice Guidelines on the Treatment of Ethylene Glycol Poisoning. Ad Hoc Committee. *J Toxicol Clin Toxcicol* 1999; 37(5):537

PROBLEM 14

An 85 year old female presents with a left hip fracture. She has been on long term calcium and vitamin D supplements as osteoporosis prophylaxis. A venous blood gas is taken and the results are shown below.

Describe and interpret the results. (100%)

FiO_2	0.21		
pH	7.49		
PO_2	43	mmHg	(5.7 kPa)
PCO_2	42	mmHg	(5.6 kPa)
HCO_3^-	32	mmol/L	
BE	+8		
O_2 Sats	78%		
Na^+	138	mmol/L	
K^+	4.7	mmol/L	
Cl^-	102	mmol/L	
PO_4^{3-}	0.5	mmol/L	
Ca^{2+}	2.8	mmol/L	
Urea	12.8	mmol/L	
Creatinine	130	μmol/L	

ANSWER

1. Acid base status

Mild alkalaemia (pH 7.49)

Normocapnoea

Moderately elevated HCO_3^-

Metabolic alkalosis

expect CO_2 = 20 + (0.7 x 32)

= 20 + 21

= 42 mmHg

therefore CO_2 is appropriate compensation

AG/DR not applicable for met alkalosis

Therefore diagnose primary metabolic alkalosis with appropriate respiratory compensation.

2. Oxygenation

Venous sample, therefore A-a gradient not applicable

3. Electrolytes

Normonatraemia
Normokalaemia

Expect K^+ for pH = 5 - (1 x 0.5) = 4.5 mmol/L
Therefore K^+ is roughly pH appropriate

Normochloraemia
Significant hypercalcaemia
Moderate hypophosphataemia
Elevated renal indices

U:C ratio ~90
Likely pre-renal

Assess volume status
Check medication history for contributors (ACEi/frusemide)

4. Interpret

VBG shows:

- Metabolic alkalosis with appropriate respiratory compensation
- Marked hypercalcaemia and hypophosphataemia
- Renal failure

Given clinical history this suggests Milk-Alkali Sx as a complication of long term Ca^{2+} therapy

- Treat IV fluids, monitor Ca^{2+}, consider diuretics/bisphosphonates
- Cease Ca^{2+} supplements
- Check ECG for QT prolongation

Other causes of high Ca^{2+}:

- Primary hyperparathyroidism
- Metastatic Ca/myeloma
  - ?pathologic fracture: evaluate xrays

Other causes alkalosis:

- Endocrinopathies
  - Cushing's Sx (less likely due to N electrolytes)
  - Bartter's Sx
  - Loop diuretics (unlikely with increased Ca/K)
  - HCl loss
    - Clarify if any vomiting

COMMENTS

An 85 year old female presents with a left hip fracture. She has been on long term calcium and vitamin D supplements as osteoporosis prophylaxis. A venous blood gas is taken and the results are shown below.

This stem again represents an unusual cue to an acid base disturbance, and candidates may wish to proceed first by systematically working the question. Doing so reveals a metabolic alkalosis complicated by hypercalcaemia and renal failure. This is the milk-alkali syndrome, caused by large amounts of calcium and ingestible alkali. Historically it was associated with milk and sodium bicarbonate treatment for peptic ulcer disease, but today is prevalent as a complication of the widespread use of calcium carbonate for osteoporosis prophylaxis[31]. Strong candidates will establish this diagnosis, as well as give a sound differential for causes of both hypercalcaemia and metabolic alkalosis as part of their interpretation.

---

31 Picolos MK, Lavis VR and Orlander PR. Milk-alkali syndrome is a major cause of hypercalcaemia among non-end-stage renal disease (non-ESRD) inpatients. *Clin Endocrinol* 2005; 63(5): 566 - 76

PROBLEM 15

A 30 year old woman presents to ED after taking an overdose of an unknown substance three hours previously. The ambulance officers report that she is confused and reporting ringing in her ears.

Her vital signs are:

HR	112	/min
BP	99/62	mmHg
RR	34	/min
Sats	100%	RA
T	37.8	°C
GCS	14	

Arterial blood gas analysis is shown below.

Describe and interpret the results. (100%)

FiO_2	0.21		
pH	7.60		
PO_2	115	mmHg	(15.3 kPa)
PCO_2	20	mmHg	(2.7 kPa)
HCO_3^-	18	mmol/L	
BE	-4		
O_2 Sats	100%		
Na^+	135	mmol/L	
K^+	5.8	mmol/L	
Cl^-	98	mmol/L	
Urea	4.5	mmol/L	
Creatinine	0.06	µmol/L	
Glucose	5.8	mmol/L	
Lactate	0.6	mmol/L	

ANSWER

1. Acid base status

Profound alkalaemia (pH 7.60)

Profound hypocapnoea

Respiratory alkalosis

Expect HCO_3^- for CO_2 20

Acute = 24 - (2 x 2) = 20mmHg

Chronic = 24 - 2 x 5 = 14mmHg

Mild decrease in HCO_3^-

Metabolic acidosis

Not consistent with either acute or chronic compensation for CO_2

Anion Gap

= 135 – 18 – 98

= 135 – 116

= 19 → RAGMA

Delta Ratio

= (19-12)/(24-18)

= 7/6

= ~1

Implies isolated RAGMA

Therefore diagnose:

acute respiratory alkalosis

metabolic acidosis

partly compensation

partly RAGMA

2. Oxygenation

Hyperoxaemia on RA

Secondary to gross hyperventilation

Implies central respiratory stimulation

A-a gradient FiO_2 21%

= 150 – (1.25 x 20) – 115

= 150 – 25 – 115
= 150 – 140
= 10

Expect A-a gradient 30yo female = 30/4 + 4 = 7.5 + 4 = 11.5
Not elevated
No V/Q mismatch

3. Electrolytes

Normonatraemia
 Not cause of confusion
Mild hyperkalaemia
 Expect K^+ for pH = 5 - 2 x 0.5 = 4.0 mmol/L
 K^+ level elevated when corrected for pH
  Monitor telemetry as pH corrected
Mild hypochloraemia
 Renal equilibration for RAGMA
Normoglycaemia
 Not cause for decreased GCS/confusion
 DKA unlikely
Normal lactate
 Not cause for RAGMA
Normal renal indices
 Not cause for RAGMA

4. Interpret

ABG shows
 acute primary respiratory alkalosis with hyperoxaemia and some metabolic compensation
 concurrent RAGMA

Primary respiratory alkalosis in absence of hypoxia implies central respiratory stimulation
 Most consistent with Aspirin overdose, given clinical Hx
  Also fits with RAGMA (N lactate and urea)
  Mx: alkalinize urine and IV fluid load
  Serial salicylate levels to Ax therapy
  Check paracetamol level (co-ingestant)

Consult toxicology
Psychiatry input RE suicide attempt

A-a gradient in kPa

A-a gradient FiO_2 21%
= 21 kPa – (1.25 x 2.7) – 15.3
= 21 – 3.38 – 15.3
= 2.32 kPa

Not Elevated (<2.5 kPa).

COMMENTS

A 30 year old woman presents to ED after taking an overdose of an unknown substance three hours previously. The ambulance officers report that she is confused and reporting ringing in her ears.

Again candidates are presented with an unknown overdose for working. However, again a clue is contained in the stem: the presence of tinnitus, classically a hallmark of aspirin overdose[32].

Working the question shows dual processes. There is a primary respiratory acidosis and a concurrent RAGMA with a normal lactate, which should immediately confirm the diagnosis for the candidate. This is a question which should engender a smile, because it a classic presentation of a core subject, and thus provides the opportunity for high marks.

Strong candidates will mention the lack of differentials for the RAGMA given a normal glucose and lactate. The fundamentals of aspirin overdose should be outlined. Alkalization of the urine to enhance elimination is indicated[33]. Serum levels and the Done nomogram are not useful in isolation, unlike the Rumack-Matthews nomogram for paracetamol poisoning[34]. However, consecutively falling levels indicate an adequate response to treatment.

Finally, strong candidates will again mention the need to examine for co-ingestants and seek input from the mental health service

---

32 O'Malley, GF. Emergency department management of the salicylate-poisoned patient. *Emerg Med Clin North Am* 2007; 25(2):333-46

33 Proudfoot AT, Krenzelok EP and Vale JA. Position paper on urine alkalinization. *J Toxicol Clin Toxicol* 2004; 42(1):1-26

34 Dugandzic RM, Tierney MG, Dickinson GE, Dolan MC and McKinght DR. Evaluation of the validity of the Done nomogram in the management of acute salicylate intoxication. *Ann Emerg Med* 1989; 18(11):1186 - 90

THE HARDER PROBLEMS

"Don't panic"
Douglas Adams

PROBLEM 16

A 26 year old asthmatic with a history of ICU admissions presents to your department in acute respiratory distress. She has been treated by her GP for 2 days with bronchodilators and glucocorticoids. Her vital signs on arrival are:

HR	120	/min
BP	110/70	mmHg
RR	30	/min
Sats	92%	40% O_2
T	37.2	^{o}C

Arterial blood gas analysis is undertaken in the resuscitation area.

Describe and interpret the results. (100%)

FiO_2	0.4		
pH	7.32		
PO_2	65	mmHg	(8.7 kPa)
PCO_2	48	mmHg	(6.4 kPa)
HCO_3^-	18	mmol/L	
BE	-6		
O_2 Sats	92%		
Na^+	142	mmol/L	
K^+	3.2	mmol/L	
Cl^-	105	mmol/L	
Glucose	10.2	mmol/L	
Lactate	3.6	mmol/L	

ANSWER

1. Acid base status

Mild acidaemia (pH 7.32)

Mild hypercapnoea

Respiratory acidosis

Expect HCO_3^- for CO_2 48

Acute = 24 + 1 = 25mmHg

Chronic = 24 + 4 = 28mmHg

Mild decrease in HCO_3^-

Metabolic acidosis

expect CO_2 = 8 + (1.5 x 18)

= 8 + 27

= 35 mmHg

Anion Gap

= 142 – 18 – 105

= 142 – 123

= 19 → RAGMA

Delta Ratio

= (19 – 12)/(24 – 18)

= 7/6

= 1

Implies isolated RAGMA

Therefore diagnose dual disturbance: primary respiratory acidosis and metabolic acidosis. No compensation.

2. Oxygenation

Critical hypoxia on supplemental oxygen.

A-a gradient FiO_2 40%

= 300 – (1.25 x 48) – 65

= 300 – 60 – 65

= 300 – 125

= 175

Grossly elevated ! (expect for 26yo female = 26/4 + 4 = ~10)

Gross V/Q mismatch
- Implies critical/life threatening asthma
- Also consider
  - ARDS (SIRS/aspiration)
  - Interstitial lung disease
  - Other respiratory membrane disease (eg LRTI)
  - PE

3. Electrolytes

Normonatraemia
Mild hypokalaemia
- Possible intracellular shift if using salbutamol
- Expect K^+ for pH = 5 + 0.5 x 0.8 = 5.4 mmol/L
- Therefore significantly K^+ deficient on correction
- Replace K^+ and monitor ECG

Normochloraemia
Moderate hyperglycaemia
- Secondary to glucocorticoid administration
- Possible diabetes – check medical Hx

Moderate hyperlactataemia
- Likely due to salbutamol administration (B_2)
- Type A less likely with normal haemodynamics
- Type B_1 less likely with N temperature, but evaluate for sepsis

4. Interpret

This is a critically ill patient*

Asthmatic, and ABG shows the dual processes of
- Respiratory acidosis
- RAGMA

Respiratory acidosis
- VERY concerning given Hx of asthma
  - Indicates critical/life threatening disease

Hypercapnoeic asthma often precedes respiratory arrest
Needs urgent treatment
High dose bronchodilators, $MgSO_4$, CPAP, possible IPPV
Involve intensive care service

RAGMA
Hyperlactataemic
Salbutamol
Sepsis/shock less likely
Check to exclude other drug causes (Iron, isoniazid, paraldehyde, toxic alcohols, metformin etc)
Also consider other causes
Diabetic ketoacidosis
Hyperglycemic: check med Hx and urine/blood ketones
Uraemia
Check renal function

A-a gradient in kPa

A-a gradient FiO_2 40%
= 40 kPa – (1.25 x 6.4) – 8.7
= 40 – 8 – 8.7
= 23.3 kPa

Grossly elevated (>2.5 kPa).

COMMENTS

A 26 year old asthmatic with a history of ICU admissions presents to your department in acute respiratory distress. She has been treated by her GP for 2 days with bronchodilators and glucocorticoids.

The stem again provides valuable information. This is a high risk patient[35], and candidates will need to add perspective to their answer.

Usually asthmatics present with hyperventilatory hypocapnoea. Here the presence of hypercarbia indicates severe asthma, and a PEFR <25% of the patient's norm[36]. Respiratory collapse is imminent. This is underlined by a comment during the evaluation of the A-a gradient to show the candidate's understanding of severity.

Several minor issues require comment in this blood gas, including the presence of a significant K^+ deficit, hyperglycaemia (presumably related to steroids) and hyperlactataemia (salbutamol therapy). Again these are included in the main body of working, so that the interpretation phase can be focused on the major issues.

Critically, in the interpretation phase the candidate must highlight the importance of the presentation. Phrases such as "this is a critically ill patient" are useful in this instance. An overview of relevant treatment is indicated. A full differential for the RAGMA can also be included should time allow.

---

35 Dhuper S, Maggiore D, Chung V and Shim C. Profile of near-fatal asthma in an inner-city hospital. *Chest* 2003; 124(5): 1880-84

36 Martin TG, Elenbaas RM and Pingleton SH. Use of peak expiratory flow rates to eliminate unnecessary arterial blood gases in acute asthma. *Ann Emerg Med* 1982 11(2):70

PROBLEM 17

A 3 year old boy presents with his parents after ingesting an unknown amount of iron tablets earlier in the day. He is vomiting profusely.

His venous blood gas is shown below.

Describe and interpret the results. (100%)

FiO_2	0.21		
pH	7.16		
PO_2	65	mmHg	(8.66 kPa)
PCO_2	25	mmHg	(3.3 kPa)
HCO_3^-	10	mmol/L	
BE	- 8		
O_2 Sats	100%		
Na^+	146	mmol/L	
K^+	6.0	mmol/L	
Cl^-	90	mmol/L	
Urea	4	mmol/L	
Creatinine	70	μmol/L	
Lactate	5.6	mmol/L	
Glucose	5.4	mmol/L	

ANSWER

1. Acid base status

Significant acidaemia (pH 7.16)

Moderate hypocapnoea

respiratory alkalosis

Significantly low bicarbonate

Moderate - severe metabolic acidosis

expect CO_2 = 8 + (1.5 x 10)

= 23mmHg

appropriate respiratory compensation

Anion Gap

= 146 – 10 – 90

= 46 → RAGMA

Delta Ratio = (46 – 12)/(24-10)

= 34/14

>2 .: Dx co-existent metabolic acidosis and metabolic alkalosis

Explains discrepancy of BE –8 for HCO_3^- 10

Therefore diagnose RAGMA, concurrent metabolic alkalosis and compensatory respiratory alkalsosis.

2. Oxygenation

pO_2 : venous sample

cannot interpret A-a gradient

3. Electrolytes

Normonatraemia

Moderate hyperkalaemia

note K^+ mildly high (6.0)

for pH 7.16 expect 5.0 + (2.5 x 0.5) = 6.25mmol/L

K^+ roughly appropriate for pH

watch and replace k as pH corrected

Mild hypochloraemia

electrical equilibrium/renal excretion RAGMA

possible HCl loss from vomiting

Normal BSL

DKA unlikely

Normal renal indices

not cause for acidosis

no renal failure complicating Fe^{3+} ingestion

Moderate hyperlactataemia

Likely cause RAGMA:

Type A - tissue hypoxia : consider hypo-perfusion secondary shock/hypotension secondary vomiting

Check volume status

Type B_1 sepsis/underlying disease (eg liver)

Type B_2 drug OD

Consistent with significant Fe^{3+} OD

Other drugs (metformin, isoniazid etc also possible)

Type B_3: inborn error of metabolism unlikely at this age

4. Interpret

3yo child: weight 14kg

60mg/kg = risk serious toxicity

VBG shows findings consistent with Fe overdose:

Lactic acidosis

Appropriate respiratory compensation

Needs quantification of dose ingested

Historical: qualify type of Fe tabs

Radiographic

Iron levels

Desferrioxamine indicated (15mg/kg IVI titrated to *vin-rose urine*). Dialysis if develops renal failure.

Also metabolic alkalosis

HCl loss from vomiting

Possible co-ingestant (eg frusemide tabs)

Paediatric presentation

- Disclosure to parents
- Evaluate for NAI/neglect

COMMENTS

A 3 year old boy presents with his parents after ingesting an unknown amount of iron tablets earlier in the day. He is vomiting profusely.

Here candidates are given the diagnosis, and some background knowledge of iron toxicity will be required. A minimum diagnosis of a RAGMA should be sought.

Working this question reveals the issue is somewhat more complex. There is a triple acid-base disturbance. The key to identifying it is to take a systematic approach and work methodically through the CO_2 level, anion gap and delta ratio. Above all, when faced with a triple disturbance candidates should not panic. RAGMA and respiratory compensation fit with acute iron overdose. Profound hypochloraemia (mathematically driving up the AG in relation to the DR) reveals a concurrent metabolic alkalosis, most likely caused by HCl loss from vomiting. Returning to the information provided in the stem validates this theory. Other differentials (co-ingestant of a loop diuretic) can be inserted as they are thought of.

As this is a paediatric presentation the usual paediatric filters should apply. Although the formulation of iron preparations varies toxicity is likely at a dose >60mg/kg elemental iron ingested [37]. NAI and parental disclosure should be mentioned in all paediatric cases.

Indications for desferrioxamine include severe systemic compromise, presence of a RAGMA, iron levels above 90mcg/mL or abdominal xray showing a large number of ingested pills (iron tablets are radiopaque)[38]. In patients with renal failure dialysis can be used to remove the chelated molecules[39].

37 Morris CC. Pediatric iron poisonings in the United States. *South Med J* 2000; 93(4):352 – 8

38 Madiwale T, Liebelt E. Iron: not a benign therapeutic drug. *Curr Opin Pediatrics* 2006; 18(2): 174-9

39 Carlsson M, Cortes D and Kanstrup T. Severe iron intoxication treated with exchange transfusion. *Arch Dis Child* 2008; 93(4):321-2

PROBLEM 18

A 68 year old diabetic woman presents with respiratory distress and severe thirst after a recent diarrhoeal illness. He daughter reports that her mother is on oral hypoglycaemics only. Her vital signs are:

HR	125	/min
BP	90/60	mmHg
RR	38	/min
Sats	99%	RA
T	37.8	°C

Her ABG from the resuscitation area is shown below.

Describe and interpret the results. (100%)

FiO_2	0.21		
pH	6.98		
PO_2	119	mmHg	(15.8 kPa)
PCO_2	14	mmHg	(1.9 kPa)
HCO_3^-	3	mmol/L	
BE	- 21		
O_2 Sats	100%		
Na^+	138	mmol/L	
K^+	7.0	mmol/L	
Cl^-	114	mmol/L	
Urea	16.4	mmol/L	
Creatinine	150	µmol/L	
Lactate	8.6	mmol/L	
Glucose	11.4	mmol/L	

ANSWER

1. Acid base status

Life threatening acidaemia (pH 6.98)
Critical hypocapnoea
Dx respiratory alkalosis

Critically low bicarbonate
Critical metabolic acidosis
expect CO_2 = 8 + (1.5 x 3)
= 12.5 mmHg
.: slight under respiratory compensation
At this HCO_3^- physiologic limits are approached

Anion Gap
= 138 – 3 – 114
= 21 → RAGMA
Delta Ratio
= (21-12)/(24-3)
= 9/21
= 0.5 .: Dx combined RAGMA and NAGMA

Therefore diagnose combined NAGMA/RAGMA and partially compensatory respiratory alkalosis.

2. Oxygenation

pO_2 → mild hyperoxia
possibly secondary to elevated RR

A-a gradient for FiO2 21%
= 150 – (1.25 x 14) – 119
= 150 – 17 – 119
= 150 – 136
= 14
Expect for 68yo female 68/4 + 4 = 17 + 4 = 21
.: Dx N A-a gradient
No V/Q mismatch exists

3. Electrolytes

Normonatraemia

Corrected for BSL = 138 + (11.4 – 5)/3
= 138 + 6/3 = 138 + 2
= 140mmol/L

Critical hyperkalaemia

Check ECG

for pH 6.98 expect 5.0 + (4.0 x 0.5) = 7.0mmol/L

K^+ roughly appropriate for pH

watch K^+ as pH corrected

Normochloraemia

Mildly elevated BSL

DKA possibly but less likely

(NB Not on insulin)

Abnormal renal indices

Both grossly elevated

U:C ratio ~100

Implies pre-renal failure

May contribute to NAGMA

Possible complication of

Diarrhoeal illness

Diabetes

Medication

Note Metformin is renally excreted

Moderate hyperlactataemia

Likely cause of RAGMA:

Type A - tissue hypoxia : consider hypo-perfusion secondary shock/hypotension due vomiting

Type B_1 sepsis/underlying disease (eg liver)

Low grade Temperature

Type B_2 drug OD

Consistent with metformin toxicity secondary to renal failure

Other drugs also possible

4. Interpret

ABG shows:

- Critical Lactic acidosis (RAGMA)
    - Needs evaluation for cause
        - Septic screen
        - Check drug history RE metformin.

- Renal failure (NAGMA)
    - Complicated by profound acidaemia
    - Haemodialysis may be indicated
    - In view of hypotension requires fluid load
        - Resuscitate to cap refill 2 secs/CVP 10mmHg
        - IDC and monitor UO
    - Evaluate for other causes of NAGMA (endocrinopathy, HCO_3^- loss due to diarrhoea)

- Hyperkalaemia
    - Likely pH and renal failure related
    - Telemetry
    - Start insulin infusion RE increased BSL and K^+

Critically ill patient, guarded prognosis
- Involve treating physicians
- ICU consult

A-a gradient in kPa

A-a gradient FiO_2 21%
= 21 kPa – (1.25 x 1.9) – 15.8
= 21 – 2.5 – 15.8
= 2.7

Not elevated for age (<4.0 kPa).

COMMENTS

A 68 year old diabetic woman presents with respiratory distress and severe thirst after a recent diarrhoeal illness. He daughter reports that her mother is on oral hypoglycaemics only.

This stem provides a large number of possibilities but no definitive guide as to the pathology underlying the arterial blood gas given.

Adequate candidates will be able to work through and define a mixed metabolic acidosis (RAGMA and NAGMA) with respiratory compensation. They can then proceed to give a list of differentials for the disorders and score a solid mark. Even though this question is of a slightly occult nature, and demonstrates multiple acid-base abnormalities, a systematic approach again will allow significant accumulation of marks.

Higher level candidates will recognise potential metformin toxicity in the context of acute renal failure. The cue here is the mention of oral hypoglycaemics in the stem of the question. Metformin is renally excreted and thus will accumulate with a resultant lactic acidosis[40]. Because it has a small volume of distribution it will be removed by dialysis.

---

40 Graham GG, Punt J, Arora M, Day RO, Doogue MP, Duong JK et al. Clinical pharmacokinetics of metformin. *Clin Pharmacokinet* 2011 50(2):81-98

PROBLEM 19.

A 65 year old long term smoker presents via the ambulance with fevers and dyspnoea. His observations are:

HR	105	/min
BP	90/60	mmHg
RR	32	/min
Sats	89%	28% O_2
T	38.5	°C

A blood gas is performed.

Describe and interpret the results. (100%)

FiO_2	0.28		
pH	7.20		
PO_2	66	mmHg	(8.8 kPa)
PCO_2	68	mmHg	(9 kPa)
HCO_3^-	20	mmol/L	
BE	+4		
Na^+	145	mmol/L	
K^+	6.0	mmol/L	
Cl^-	100	mmol/L	
Urea	12	mmol/L	
Creatinine	100	µmol/L	
Lactate	2.6	mmol/L	

ANSWER

1. Acid-Base Balance

Moderate acidaemia

Significant hypercapnoea

Respiratory acidosis

expect HCO_3^-:

acute to be 24 + 3 = 27mmol/L

chronically to be 24 + (4 x 3) = 36mmol/L

Mild decrease HCO_3^-

Metabolic Acidosis

Expect CO_2 = 8 + 1.5 x 20

= 38mmH

Anion Gap

= 145 – 20 – 100

= 25

Delta Ratio

= (25 – 12)/(24 – 20)

= 13/4 = 3.25

Implies pre-extant or co-extant metabolic alkalosis

Therefore diagnose triple disturbance of respiratory acidosis, metabolic acidosis and metabolic alkalosis (likely compensation for chronic CO_2 retention)

2. Oxygenation

Significantly hypoxic

A-a gradient FiO_2 28%

= 200 – (1.25 x 68) – 66

= 200 – 85 – 66

= 200 – 151

= 49

Expect 65yo man A-a = 65/4 + 4 = 20

Raised A-a grad implies V/Q Mismatch

LRTI/APO

ARDS
Chronic resp membrane disease
PE

3. Electrolytes

Normonatraemia
Mild hyperkalaemia
For pH 7.20 expect $K^+ = 5.0 + (2 \times 0.5) = 6.0$mmol/L
K^+ appropriate for pH
Normochloraemia
Mild elevation of renal indices
U:C ratio > 100
Implies pre-renal failure
Mild hyperlactataemia (<4.0mmol/L)
Type A – dehydration/hypo-perfusion (renal failure)
Type B_1 – sepsis (febrile)
Type B_2 – check medications (metformin, iron etc)

4. Interpet

Critically ill patient
Respiratory acidosis
Likely acute on chronic given co-extant metabolic alkalosis
Smoker – likely COPD
BiPAP indicated until resolution of acute fraction of respiratory acidosis
RAGMA plus high lactate
Resuscitate, fluids, bronchodilators, steroids if wheezy
Broad spectrum ABx
Needs full septic screen
Metabolic alkalosis
Likely chronic if Hx COAD
Consider other causes eg loop diuretics

A-a gradient in kPa

A-a gradient FiO_2 28%
= 28 kPa – (1.25 x 9) – 8.8
= 28 – 11.25 – 8.8
= 7.95

Elevated (>2.5 kPa).

COMMENTS

A 65 year old long term smoker presents via the ambulance with fevers and dyspnoea.

Although this question may seem very convoluted, with a triple acid-base disturbance, it illustrates the importance of noting the clues given in the stem. In a long term smoker with fever, dyspnoea and hypotension the obvious picture is one of an infective exacerbation of COPD.

The key to understanding the triple disturbance is the delta-ratio of >2.0. In other words the fall in anion gap has been more than twice the fall in bicarbonate expected. The implication is of a pre-extant metabolic alkalosis, most likely in a smoker as part of the picture of chronic type II respiratory failure. Good candidates might mention another possibility for the metabolic alkalosis (in this case the use of diuretics) to show completeness of knowledge.

Neither pH nor HCO_3^- correct for each other, and this makes it very difficult to delineate the exact degree of acute respiratory acidosis. The co-existing metabolic alkalosis however makes it quite likely that there is an element of chronic CO_2 retention.

Finally, to draw a line under the clinical information given, a good candidate will mention administration of medical therapy and a trial of bilevel non invasive ventilation, which has a treatment benefit for these patients[41].

41 Ram FS, Picot J, Lightowler J and Wedzicha JA, Non-invasive positive pressure ventilation for treatment of respiratory failure due to exacerbations of chronic obstructive pulmonary disease. *Cochrane Database Syst Rev*. 2004.

PROBLEM 20

Your intern asks you to a review a patient in the short stay ward. She is a 26 year old previously well woman, admitted with dehydration because of gastroenteritis. Overnight she has had 6L of 0.9% NaCl, and she is now complaining of dyspnoea and orthopnoea.

Her ABG results are shown below.

Describe and interpret the results. (70%)

Outline your further actions. (30%)

FiO_2	0.21		
pH	7.15		
PO_2	62	mmHg	(8.26 kPa)
PCO_2	50	mmHg	(6.7 kPa)
HCO_3^-	16	mmol/L	
BE	-8		
O_2 Sats	91%		
Na^+	151	mmol/L	
K^+	5.2	mmol/L	
Cl^-	126	mmol/L	
Urea	5.7	mmol/L	
Creatinine	60	µmol/L	

ANSWER

1. Acid base status

Moderate acidaemia (pH 7.15)

Hypercapnoea
Respiratory acidosis
Expect HCO_3^- for CO_2 50:
Acute = 24 + (1 x 1) = 25
Chronic = 24 + (1 x 4) = 29
Moderately low bicarbonate
Metabolic acidosis
expect CO_2 = 8 + 1.5 x 16
= 32 mmHg
Anion Gap
= 151 – 16 – 126
= 151 – 142
= 9 → NAGMA
Delta Ratio
= (9-12)/(24-16)
= <0
.: Dx isolated NAGMA
Fits with BE –8 for HCO_3^- 16

Therefore diagnose dual process: combined respiratory acidosis and NAGMA.

2. Oxygenation

pO_2 → significant hypoxia on RA
needs supplemental O2

A-a gradient FiO_2 21%
= 150 – (1.25 x 50) – 62
= 150 – 62 – 62
= 150 – 124
= 26

Expect for 26yo female 26/4 + 4 = 4.5 + 4 = 8.5

.: Dx elevated A-a gradient → Dx V/Q mismatch
Concerning for APO given Hx of large volume crystalloid
ARDS (SIRS/aspiration)
Interstitial lung disease
Other respiratory membrane disease (eg LRTI)
PE

3. Electrolytes

Mild hypernatraemia
Secondary Na^+ load
Mild hyperkalaemia
for pH 7.15 expect 5.0 + (1.5 x 0.5) = 5.75mmol/L
.: K^+ very mildly low for pH
watch K^+ as pH corrected
Hyperchloraemia
NAGMA
Cl load from NaCl

Renal indices normal
No evidence pre-renal failure

4. Interpret

ABG shows:
Combined respiratory acidosis, V/Q mismatch and NAGMA

Respiratory acidosis + V/Q mismatch
Iatrogenic APO (8L crystalloid!)
Other pulmonary disease
Pneumonia
PE
ARDS
Needs CXR and evaluation for same

NAGMA
Likely iatrogenic – excessive NaCl administration
Other causes:
Drugs – acetazolamide, spironolactone

Addison's – less likely given elevated Na^+
Renal failure unlikely with N indices

Therefore based on above, further actions are:

Ix and Rx patient
CXR, volume status Ax, septic screen if warranted
Treat APO – CPAP, diuresis, supplemental O_2
Arrange admission

Iatrogenic error
Investigate systems/process/individual
Educate staff – individuals, review at M+M
Apologize to patient: full and open disclosure
Documentation of same
Manage risk : brief director, medicolegal organization

Ongoing quality assurance and feedback for any changes made

A-a gradient in kPa

A-a gradient FiO_2 21%
= 21 kPa – (1.25 x 6.7) – 8.26
= 21 – 8.37 – 8.26
= 4.37

Elevated (>2.5 kPa).

COMMENTS

Your intern asks you to a review a patient in the short stay ward. She is a 26 year old previously well woman, admitted with dehydration because of gastroenteritis. Overnight she has had 6 litres of 0.9% NaCl, and she is now complaining of dyspnoea and orthopnoea.

Her ABG results are shown below.

Describe and interpret the results (70%)
Outline your further actions (30%)

This question exemplifies a hard VAQ, because it occurs in two parts. Time pressure may be an issue. Candidates are asked to describe and interpret, as well as outline their further actions. However, the presence of a second part to the question asking for further actions should reassure candidates. It implies that the ABG will be diagnostic, as there are specific details the examiners will subsequently look for. Often the "part B" of a question is a natural extension of the interpretation phase of the question.

Here, the stem clearly suggests iatrogenic pulmonary oedema. Normal saline has a pH of around 5.5[42] and will result in a NAGMA if administered in excessive amount. Thus candidates could expect acute pulmonary oedema manifesting as respiratory acidosis with an elevated A-a gradient, and possibly a NAGMA. It is important, as always, to mention a list of relevant differentials.

When answering a question asking for an outline of further actions, broad brush subject headings are very helpful. In this case a consultant would ensure the welfare of the patient, manage an iatrogenic error, apologize to the patient and evaluate the ED system to ensure the error does not recur.

42 Reddi B. Why is saline so acidic (and does it really matter?). *Int J Med Sci* 2013; 10(6): 747 - 750

PROBLEM 21

A 16 year old girl presents with her parents with thirst and dyspnoea. Her parents report periods of excessive vomiting over the last six days, accompanied by significant weight loss. Her BMI is 16.

Her venous blood gas is shown below.

Describe and interpret the results. (100%)

FiO_2	0.21		
pH	7.42		
PO_2	98	mmHg	(13.0 kPa)
PCO_2	35	mmHg	(4.7 kPa)
HCO_3^-	18	mmol/L	
BE	+6		
O_2 Sats	99%		
Na^+	138	mmol/L	
K^+	2.8	mmol/L	
Cl^-	66	mmol/L	
Mg^+	0.7	mmol/L	
PO_4^{3-}	0.5	mmol/L	
Albumin	28	g/L	
Glucose	5.4	mmol/L	
Urea	1.2	mmol/L	
Creatinine	32	µmol/L	
Lactate	0.6mmol/L		

ANSWER

1. Acid base status

pH normal – not acidaemic or alkalaemic

Normocapnoea

Mildly decreased HCO_3^-

Metabolic acidosis

expect CO_2 = 8 + (1.5 x 18)
= 8 + 27
= 35 mmHg

therefore CO_2 is appropriate respiratory compensation

Anion Gap
= 138 – 18 – 66
= 138 – 84
= 54 → RAGMA

Delta Ratio
= (54 – 12)/(24-18)
= 42/6
= 7

Identifies concurrent metabolic alkalosis occurring
Explains discrepancy between BE +6 and HCO_3^- 18

Therefore diagnose mixed metabolic picture: RAGMA and metabolic alkalosis occurring concurrently

2. Oxygenation

VBG – cannot interpret oxygenation status

3. Electrolytes

Normonatraemia

Mild- moderate hypokalaemia

No correction for pH

Critical hypochloraemia

Renal excretion or GIT loss (vomiting)

Mild hypomagnesaemia

Nutritional/renal loss

Moderate hypophosphataemia

May be nutritional or due to hyperventilation

Moderate hypoalbuminaemia

Broad DDx: nutrition, inflammation, oedema, ca

Markedly decreased renal indices

Poor muscle mass (BMI 16)

Decreased production of metabolites

Normoglycaemia

DKA unlikely as cause of RAGMA

Normal lactate

Unlikely to be cause of RAGMA

4. Interpret

ABG shows:

Mixed RAGMA and alkalosis

Multiple electrolyte abnormalities: low K^+, Mg^+, PO_4^{3-}

Evidence of malnutrition/low muscle bulk

Clinical Hx implies significant eating disorder

Anorexia Nervosa/Bulimia Nervosa

Complicated by:

RAGMA

Possible starvation ketoacidosis

Check urinary/blood ketones

Other causes less likely with N glucose, renal indices and lactate. If evidence sepsis perform septic screen

Metabolic alkalosis

Loss of HCl secondary vomiting

Explains critical hypochloraemia

Also consider diuretic abuse, endocrinopathies

- Electrolyte abnormalities
  - High risk refeeding syndrome
  - Need prophylactic replacement and cardiac monitoring
  - Can confirm malnutrition with pre-albumin assay

Requires admission

- Full disclosure to parents
- Involve ICU, psychiatry, eating disorders unit

COMMENTS

A 16 year old girl presents with her parents with thirst and dyspnoea. Her parents report periods of excessive vomiting over the last six days, accompanied by significant weight loss. Her BMI is 16.

The stem provided to candidates gives a strong indicator that the patient has an eating disorder. Starvation ketoacidosis is a rare but important cause of RAGMA, and is often accompanied by multiple electrolyte abnormalities[43]. The role of excessive HCl loss with a resultant metabolic alkalosis has already been discussed. Here it explains the widely distorted delta ratio.

Hypoalbuminaemia and low plasma creatinine may be reflective of decreased muscle bulk (as well as many other pathologies). The hallmark of refeeding syndrome is hypophosphataemia and this may cause acute respiratory failure. Thus early replacement of all major electrolytes is warranted.

Strong candidates will again note the role of other services in this patient's care, particularly the need for the involvement of an eating disorder psychiatrist. Other differentials for the major metabolic findings should also be mentioned.

43 NiBhraonain S and Lawton L. Chronic malnutrition may in fact be an acute emergency. *J Emerg Med* 2013; 44: 72-4

PROBLEM 22

A 65 year old female with a history of bowel resection for colorectal cancer presents to the emergency room with a distended, painful abdomen and profuse vomiting.

Her vital signs are:

HR	120	/min
BP	99/55	mmHg
RR	22	/min
Sats	92%	40% O_2
T	38.7	°C

Her arterial blood gas is shown below.

Describe and interpret the results. (100%)

FiO_2	0.40		
pH	7.46		
PO_2	66	mmHg	(8.8 kPa)
PCO_2	68	mmHg	(9.0 kPa)
HCO_3^-	37	mmol/L	
BE	+12		
O_2 Sats	92%		
Na^+	138	mmol/L	
K^+	4.8	mmol/L	
Cl^-	72	mmol/L	
Lactate	1.2	mmol/L	
Glucose	2.6	mmol/L	

ANSWER

1. Acid base status

Mild alkalaemia (pH 7.46)

Hypercapnoea
Respiratory acidosis

Significantly elevated HCO_3^-
Metabolic alkalosis
expect CO_2 = 20 + (0.7 x 37)
= 20 + 27
= 47 mmHg
therefore CO_2 is more than expected as appropriate compensation
AG/DR not applicable for met alkalosis

Therefore diagnose primary metabolic alkalosis, and concurrent (non compensatory) respiratory acidosis

2. Oxygenation

Critically hypoxic on supplemental oxygen

A-a gradient FiO_2 40%
= 300 – (1.25 x 68) – 66
= 300 – 85 – 66
= 300 – 151
= 149

Expect A-a gradient 65yo female = 65/4 + 4 = 16 + 4 = 20

Dx raised A-a gradient and V/Q mismatch
ARDS (SIRS/aspiration) due to vomiting
Interstitial lung disease
Other respiratory membrane disease (eg LRTI/APO)
PE

3. Electrolytes

Normonatraemia
Normokalaemia
    Expect K^+ for pH = 5 - (0.5 x 0.6) = 5 – 0.3 = 4.70 mmol/L
    Therefore K^+ is pH appropriate
Profound hypochloraemia
    GIT loss due to vomiting
Significant hypoglycaemia
    Needs correction with 50ml 50% dextrose IV
Normal lactate
    Severe sepsis/mesenteric ischaemia less likely

4. Interpret

ABG shows:
    Metabolic alkalosis and respiratory acidosis as two distinct entities

Metabolic alkalosis
    Hypochloraemic
    Hx vomiting and surgery – implies bowel obstruction with HCl loss
    Also evaluate other causes
        Bartter's/Cushing's syndrome
        Drugs: loop diuretics
        Milk-alkali syndrome

Respiratory acidosis and hypoxia
    Type II respiratory failure
    V/Q mismatch – given fever, and Hx vomiting concern RE aspiration
        CXR
        Early treatment for aspiration LRTI
        Search for other causes: BC x 2 and Urine m/c/s
        Other causes of V/Q mismatch as mentioned earlier
        CTPA if clinically indicated to exclude PE

Needs treatment for bowel obstruction + LRTI
    IV fluid titrated to HR < 100 and SBP > 100mmHg
    Abx for source of sepsis

IDC, surgical input plus AXR or CT abdomen
Analgesia/antiemetics
Replace glucose

A-a gradient in kPa

A-a gradient FiO_2 40%
$= 40\ kPa - (1.25 \times 8.8) - 9.0$
$= 40 - 11.0 - 9.0$
$= 20$

Grossly elevated (>2.5 kPa).

COMMENTS

A 65 year old female with a history of bowel resection for colorectal cancer presents to the emergency room with a distended, painful abdomen and profuse vomiting.

This question represents a double acid base disturbance of metabolic alkalosis and respiratory acidosis. The respiratory acidosis is more severe than would be expected as calculated compensation, and thus (in conjunction with a raised A-a gradient) is likely to represent independent pathology. Strong candidates will describe both abnormalities with appropriate differential diagnoses, and then link them back to the clinical cues provided in the stem. It is highly likely this lady has a bowel obstruction with vomiting complicated by HCl loss and aspiration.

Again, working through the question in a systematic fashion is key to achieving a high mark.

PROBLEM 23

A 60 year old patient presents to ED with pleuritic chest pain and haemoptysis. He has a history of DVT three years ago and is currently on aspirin.

His vital signs are:

HR	135	/min
BP	82/45	mmHg
RR	39	/min
Sats	88%	15L NRB
T	36.8	°C

Urgent arterial blood gas analysis is shown below.

Describe and interpret the results. (100%)

FiO_2	0.6		
pH	7.10		
PO_2	55	mmHg	(7.3 kPa)
PCO_2	55	mmHg	(7.3 kPa)
HCO_3^-	16	mmol/L	
BE	-8		
O_2 Sats	88%		
Na^+	139	mmol/L	
K^+	6.0	mmol/L	
Cl^-	103	mmol/L	
Lactate	8.7	mmol/L	

ANSWER

1. Acid base status

Profound acidaemia (pH 7.10)

Moderate hypercapnoea

Respiratory acidosis

Expect HCO_3^- for CO_2 60

Acute = 24 + 2 = 26mmHg

Chronic = 24 + 8 = 32mmHg

Moderate decrease in HCO_3^-

Metabolic acidosis

expect CO_2 = 8 + (1.5 x 16)

= 8 + 24

= 32 mmHg

Anion Gap

= 139 – 16 – 103

= 139 – 119

= 20 → RAGMA

Delta Ratio

= (20 – 12)/(24 – 16)

= 8/8

= 1

Implies isolated RAGMA

Therefore diagnose dual disturbance: primary respiratory acidosis and metabolic acidosis. No compensation.

2. Oxygenation

Life threatening hypoxia on supplemental oxygen.

A-a gradient FiO_2 60%

= 450 – (1.25 x 60) – 55

= 450 – 75 – 55

= 450 – 130

= 320

Grossly elevated!

expect for 60yo male = 60/4 + 4 = 19

Gross V/Q mismatch

Given Hx and haemodynamic instability implies massive PE

Also consider

ARDS (SIRS/aspiration)

Interstitial lung disease

Other respiratory membrane disease (eg LRTI, APO)

3. Electrolytes

Normonatraemia

Mild hyperkalaemia

Expect K^+ for pH = 5 + (3 x 0.5) = 6.5 mmol/L

Actually mildly hypokalaemic for pH

Monitor K^+ as pH corrected

Normochloraemia

Significant hyperlactataemia

Probably type A: gross tissue hypo perfusion (obstructive shock)

Other causes

Type B_1 – sepsis, liver failure (less likely given Hx)

Type B_2 – drugs (salbutamol, isoniazid, iron, paraldehyde, toxic alcohols etc)

4. Interpret

This is a critically ill patient*

ABG shows the dual processes of

Respiratory acidosis with profound V/Q mismatch

RAGMA + hyperlactaemia

Implies massive PE, haemodynamically unstable patient, peri-arrest

May be too unstable for CTPA or ECHO

Indication for urgent thrombolysis (or embolectomy)

Informed consent if possible

Notify respiratory medicine/Cardiothoracic Surgery urgently

Clinically/radiographically (mobile CXR/FAST-E) exclude tension Ptx and tamponade as causes of obstructive shock prior to lysis
ECG – evaluate for R heart strain/arrhythmia
ECHO could be used to confirm R heart strain prior to lysis

Causes of V/Q mismatch as noted earlier. Evaluate for these.

Other causes of RAGMA to consider (much less likely in this patient)

- Diabetic ketoacidosis
  - Check BSL/med Hx
- Uraemia
  - Check renal function

A-a gradient in kPa

A-a gradient FiO_2 60%
= 60 kPa – (1.25 x 7.3) – 7.3
= 60 – 9.13 – 7.3
= 43.57

Grossly elevated (>2.5 kPa).

COMMENTS

A 60 year old patient presents to ED with pleuritic chest pain and haemoptysis. He has a history of DVT three years ago and is currently on aspirin.

The information provides the likely diagnosis. It is highly probable that this patient has suffered an episode of pulmonary venous thromboembolism. Candidates should note the observations given in this case:

HR	*135*
BP	*82/45*
RR	*39*
Sats	*88% 15L*
T	*36.8°C*

This patient is clearly peri-arrest, and could reasonably be expected to have systemic underperfusion manifesting as a lactic acidosis. Systemic working will reveal the two independent processes occurring, namely respiratory acidosis with a massive A-a gradient and a RAGMA, but the key here is to show perspective. The patient is critically ill, and there are multiple indications given for consideration of thrombolytic therapy[44]. The role of echocardiography in urgent assessment has long been established[45] and strong candidates will mention this as an important risk stratification tool. The importance of excluding other causes of obstructive shock prior to any intervention should also be made clear.

44 Goldhaber SZ. Modern treatment of pulmonary embolism. *Eur Respir J* 2003; Suppl 35:22s

45 Come PC. Echocardiographic evaluation of pulmonary embolism and its response to therapeutic interventions. *Chest* 1992; 101:151s

PROBLEM 24

A 40 year old man is brought by ambulance to your emergency department after a fire at a factory. He has no airway compromise or evidence of cutaneous burns, but he is GCS 12 and acutely confused. His blood pressure is 120/80 and his pulse oxygen saturation is 99%.

A blood gas is shown below.

Describe and interpret the results. (100%).

FiO_2	0.21		
pH	6.96		
PO_2	82	mmHg	(10.9 kPa)
PCO_2	58	mmHg	(7.7 kPa)
HCO_3^-	5	mmol/L	
BE	-19		
HbCO	26%		
O_2 Sats	91%		
Na^+	136	mmol/L	
K^+	4.0	mmol/L	
Cl^-	96	mmol/L	
Urea	5	mmol/L	
Creatinine	90	µmol/L	
Lactate	16	mmol/L	
Glucose	5.4	mmol/L	

ANSWER

1. Acid base status

Critical acidaemia (pH 6.96)

Moderate hypercapnoea
Respiratory acidosis
hypo ventilation secondary head injury/loc/seizure
HCO_3^- compensation acute should = 26mmol/L

Critically low bicarbonate and BE -19
critical metabolic acidosis
expect CO2 = 8 + (1.5 x 5)
= 15mmHg
Anion Gap
= 35
delta ratio
= (35-12)/(24-4)
= 23/19
= 1.1 (<2.0) .: isolated RAGMA

Therefore diagnose respiratory acidosis and concurrent RAGMA. Dual process, no compensation.

2. Oxygenation

pO_2 room air lower than expected but not grossly hypoxic

Pulse Sats 99% > measured sats/expected for pO2, ie saturation gap
Left shift of O_2-Hb curve
CO toxicity: HbCO level 26%
hyperbaric O_2 indicated

A-a gradient FiO2 21%
= 150 – (1.25 x 58) - 82
= 150 – 75 – 82
= -7
i.e. normal
no V/Q mismatch exists

3. Electrolytes

Normonatraemia
Normokalaemia
    note K normal but low for ph expect higher
    expect 5 + 5 x 0.5 = 7.5mmol/L
    likely full body K deficient
    watch and replace k as ph corrected
Mild hypochloraemia
    electrical equilibrium/renal excretion RAGMA

Normal BSL
    not cause for decreased gcs
Normal renal indices
    not cause for acidosis

Critical hyperlactataemia
    Likely cause RAGMA:
    Type A - tissue hypoxia : **CYANIDE** toxicity (note normoxic tissue hypoxia in setting of fire), also consider hypo-perfusion secondary shock/hypotension
    Type B_1 sepsis/underlying disease (eg liver)
    Type B_2 drug OD (salicylates, tox alcohols etc)

4. Interpret

This is a critically ill patient
    respiratory acidosis
    may need ventilatory support
RAGMA
    likely lactic with N BSL and renal indices
    carbon monoxide poisoning plus neurologic compromise
        high flow O_2 indicated
    critical lactic acidosis suggests cyanide toxicity in context of fire: empiric treatment with hydroxycobalamin and thiosulfate is indicated
Also consider other causes decreased GCS: closed head injury/trauma

A-a gradient in kPa

A-a gradient FiO_2 21%

= 21 kPa – (1.25 x 7.7) – 10.9
= 21 – 9.63 – 10.9
= 0.47

Not elevated (<2.5 kPa).

COMMENTS

A 40 year old man is brought by ambulance to your emergency department after a fire at a factory. He has no airway compromise or evidence of cutaneous burns, but he is GCS 12 and acutely confused. His blood pressure is 120/80 and his oxygen saturation is 99%.

This is a somewhat obtuse question, but the mention of a fire should raise the spectre of carbon monoxide poisoning. This is clearly evident in the elevated HbCO level given in the question. However, astute candidates will note that there is a discrepancy between the observed oxygen saturation and the calculated oxygen saturation: the so called "saturation gap". There is also a substantial difference between the measured arterial oxygen tension and tissue perfusion, as measured by an extreme lactic acidosis. In other words there is a normoxic tissue hypoxia.

The saturation gap is due to a misread from the pulse oximeter, and strongly implies the presence of an abnormal form of haemoglobin, usually HbCO. It is strongly suggestive of carbon monoxide poisoning[46]. High flow oxygen is indicated as a minimum. The indications for hyperbaric oxygen remain controversial[47] but probably apply in this case.

The phenomenon of normoxic tissue hypoxia (the presence of adequate oxygen in the tissues but the inability to metabolise it) suggests cyanide toxicity. In developed countries cyanide poisoning is most commonly

46 Akhtar J, Johnston BD and Krenzelok EP. Mind the gap. *J Emerg Med* 2007; 33(2):131-2.

47 Kao LW and Nanagas KA. Carbon monoxide poisoning. *Emerg Med Clin North Am* 2004; 22(4):985-1018

associated with fires and industrial accidents[48]. Cyanide uncouples oxidative phosphorylation and electron transport, and is therefore non responsive to conventional measures of improving oxygenation. It requires empiric treatment with one of several antidotes, most commonly hydroxocobalamin and sodium thiosulfate[31].

Strong candidates will discuss both these possibilities, as well as other differentials for the patients decreased level of consciousness, including head injury.

---

48 Megarbane B, Delahaye A, Goldgran-Toledano D and Baud FJ. Antidotal treatment of cyanide poisoning. *J Chin Med Assoc* 2003; 66(4): 193-203

PROBLEM 25

A 35 year old male multi-trauma victim attends your hospital with the ambulance service after a high speed MVA. The ambulance have given him several liters of crystalloid en route to hospital. He has obvious chest injuries.

His vital signs are:

HR	110	/min
BP	95/75	mmHg
RR	34	/min
Sats	92%	40% O^2
T	35.4	°C
GCS	7 ($E_1V_2M_4$)	

Urgent arterial blood gas analysis is undertaken and the results are shown below.

Describe and interpret them. (70%)

Outline your management priorities. (30%)

FiO_2	0.4		
pH	7.09		
PO_2	76	mmHg	(10.1 kPa)
PCO_2	65	mmHg	(8.7 kPa)
HCO_3^-	14	mmol/L	
BE	-8		
O_2 Sats	92%		
Na^+	135	mmol/L	
K^+	4.2	mmol/L	
Cl^-	103	mmol/L	
Glucose	6.2	mmol/L	
Lactate	4.1	mmol/L	
Hb	82	g/dL	

ANSWER

1. Acid base status

Severe acidaemia (pH 7.09)

Severe hypercarbia

Respiratory acidosis

Expect HCO_3^- for CO_2 65

Acute = 24 + (2.5 x 1) = 26.5mmol/L

Chronic = 24 + (2.5 x 4) = 34mmol/L

Moderate decrease in HCO_3^-

Metabolic acidosis

Expect CO_2 = 8 + (1.5 x 14)

= 8 + 21

= 29

Anion Gap

= 135 – 14 – 103

= 135 – 117

= 18 → RAGMA

Delta Ratio

= (18-12)/(24-14)

= 6/10

= 0.6

Implies concurrent NAGMA and RAGMA

Therefore diagnose triple disturbance:

acute respiratory acidosis

RAGMA

NAGMA

No compensation

2. Oxygenation

Significant hypoxaemia on supplemental O_2

A-a gradient FiO_2 40%

= 300 – (1.25 x 65) – 76

= 300 – 80 – 76

= 300 – 156
= ~144

Expect A-a gradient 35yo male = 35/4 + 4 = 9 + 4 = 13
Significant V/Q mismatch
Given Hx concern RE
Pulmonary contusion/flail segment
ARDS/SIRS
Aspiration

3. Electrolytes

Normonatraemia
Normokalaemia
Expect K^+ for pH = 5 + (2.5 x 0.5) = 6.25 mmol/L
Hypokalaemic for pH : correct as pH corrected
Normochloraemia
Normoglycaemia
Severe hyperlactataemia
Likely cause for RAGMA
Profound anaemia
Probably due to significant haemorrhage
Needs transfusion
Be prepared for massive transfusion protocol

4. Interpret

Critically injured patient: hypotensive, hypoxic, tachycardic, hypothermic, obtunded
Critical triad: hypothermic, acidotic → check coag status!

ABG shows
Respiratory acidosis
RAGMA
NAGMA

Respiratory acidosis plus raised A-a gradient
Pulmonary contusion
Haemo/pneumothorax
ARDS/APO
Other causes – fat embolism, PE, resp membrane defect

Poor prognosis if closed head injury

RAGMA

Hyperlactataemia

Hypovolaemic shock

Poor prognostic indicator

NAGMA

Excessive crystalloid administration

Renal failure

Other source HCO_3^- loss

Management priorities

Secure airway (GCS <8)

Ventilate to reverse resp acidosis

Decompress chest if required

Resuscitate: blood, massive transfusion protocol

Warm fluid

Tranexamic acid

Transfer to definitive care

OT, if stabilizes consider CT, otherwise FAST

Social worker for family

A-a gradient in kPa

A-a gradient FiO_2 40%

= 40 kPa – (1.25 x 8.7) – 10.1
= 40 – 10.87 – 10.1
= 19.03

Grossly elevated (>2.5 kPa).

COMMENTS

A 35 year old male multi-trauma victim attends your hospital with the ambulance service after a high speed MVA. The ambulance have given him several litres of crystalloid en route to hospital. He has obvious chest injuries.

His vital signs are:

HR	*110*
BP	*95/75*
RR	*34*
Sats	*92% 6L*
T	*35.4°C*
GCS	*7 ($E_1V_2M_4$)*

The stem provides a familiar scenario to experienced emergency physicians. Based on the vital signs and the cue regarding chest injuries significant disturbances of the A-a gradient should be anticipated. The association of the administration of saline with a normal anion gap acidosis has already been discussed, and hypoperfusion is an important cause of a hyperlactataemic RAGMA. Systematic working of the question will reveal all of these abnormalities without too much effort.

Strong candidates will mention some of the key issues in care of the trauma patient. The deleterious triad of acidosis, hypothermia and coagulopathy in a trauma patient is well described[49]. Key priorities will be management of the airway [50], re-warming and correction of the coagulopathy, administration of tranexamic acid[51], transfer to definitive care and care of the patient's family. As the stem only asks for an "outline" of these issues they can be dealt with using broad brush strokes and little detail.

49 Rossaint R, Cerny V, Coats TJ, Duranteau J, Fernandez-Mondejar E, Gordini G et al. Key issues in advanced bleeding care in trauma. *Shock* 2006; 26:322-31

50 Gentleman D, Deaden M, Midgelu S and Maclean D. Guidelines for resuscitation and transfer of patients with serious head injury. *BMJ* 1997; 307:547-552

51 The CRASH-2 trial collaborators. Effects of tranexamic acid on death, vascular occlusive events, and blood transfusion in trauma patients with significant haemorrhage (CRASH-2): a randomized, placebo-controlled trial. *The Lancet* 2010; 376(9734): 23 - 32

PROBLEM 26.

A 26 year old man presents to your hospital complaining of nausea and vomiting and acute visual loss in both eyes. He has just returned from a holiday in South East Asia.

His vital signs are:

HR	105	/min
BP	120/90	mmHg
RR	30	/min
Sats	92%	40% O_2
T	36.9	°C

Arterial blood gas is shown below.

Describe and interpret the results. (100%)

FiO_2	0.40		
pH	7.10		
PO_2	70	mmHg	(9.3 kPa)
PCO_2	60	mmHg	(8.0 kPa)
HCO_3^-	14	mmol/L	
BE	-8		
Na^+	136	mmol/L	
K^+	6.5	mmol/L	
Cl^-	100	mmol/L	
Urea	8.5	mmol/L	
Creatinine	100	μmol/L	
Lactate	5.8	mmol/L	
Glucose	4.5	mmol/L	
Osm_c	340	mosm/Kg	

ANSWER

1. Acid-Base Balance

Severe acidaemia

Significant hypercapnoea

Respiratory acidosis

Expect HCO_3^-:

acute = 24 + 2 = 26 mmol/L

chronic = 24 + 8 = 32 mmol/L

Moderately low bicarbonate

Metabolic acidosis

Expect pCO_2 = (8 + 1.5 x 14)

= 29mmHg

Anion Gap

= 136 - (100+14)

= 136 - 114

= 22

Delta Ratio

= (22 - 12)/(24 - 14)

= 10/10 = 1.0

Therefore diagnose isolated RAGMA

Overall picture: dual disturbance of respiratory acidosis and metabolic acidosis

2. Oxygenation

A-a gradient for FiO_2 40%

= 300 - (1.25 x 60) - 70

= 300 - 75 - 70

= 225 - 70

= 155

Expect A-a grad for 26yo man = 26/4 + 4 = 10.5mmHg

Therefore elevated A-a gradient suggests V/Q mismatch

ARDS (SIRS/aspiration)
Interstitial lung disease
Other respiratory membrane disease
PE

3. Biochemistry

Normonatraemia
Moderate hyperkalaemia
Expect K+ for pH 7.10 = 5 + (3 x 0.5) = 6.5 mmol/L
K+ level appropriate for pH
Significantly elevated lactate
Normoglycaemia
Normal renal indices
Osmolar gap
= osmm - osmc
= 340 - (2 x 136 + 4.5 + 8.5)
= 340 - (272 + 13)
= 340 - 285
= 55 elevated

4. Interpret

Critically ill man
Dual disturbance:
Resp acidosis, concern RE aspiration/ARDS
Metabolic acidosis
RAGMA + high lactate + osmolar gap
.: Likely diagnosis given Hx of visual disturbance is methanol toxicity
Critically unwell
Multiple indications for dialysis
pH <7.30
Visual changes
Check urine oxalic acid (ethylene glycol) and consider co-ingestants
Treat until dialysis with alcohol or fomepizole

A-a gradient in kPa

A-a gradient FiO_2 40%
$= 40kPa - (1.25 \times 8) - 9.3$
$= 40 - 10 - 9.3$
$= 40 - 19.3$
$= 20.7$

Elevated (>2.5 kPa).

COMMENTS

A 26 year old man presents to your hospital complaining of nausea and vomiting and acute visual loss in both eyes. He has just returned from a holiday in South East Asia.

This slightly unusual stem does not give a great deal of information to enable candidates to make an initial diagnosis.

However, when the question is worked carefully a large amount of information can be gathered to enable the stem to be interpreted. Astute candidates will notice the presence of a measured serum osmolality in the pathology results given, implying that an osmolar gap will need to be calculated. Working through the question reveals the presence of a RAGMA with hyperlactataemia and a raised osmolar gap, all of which imply the presence of a toxic alcohol[52].

Returning to the stem, the significance of the symptoms described should become obvious. Visual loss is classically a symptom of methanol poisoning[53] (among other substances), allowing a specific toxic alcohol to be specified as the poisoning agent by astute candidates. Some

---

[52] Lynd LD, Richardson KJ, Purssell RA, Abu-Laban RB, Brubacher JR, Lepik KJ et al. An evaluation of the osmole gap as a screening test for toxic alcohol poisoning. BMC Emerg Med 2008; 8:5

[53] Stelmach MZ and O'Day J. Partly reversible visual failure with methanol toxicity. *ANZ J Opthalm* 1992; 20(1) 57-64

candidates may also remember a series of well publicized reports of methanol poisoning in returned travelers in Asian resort areas[54].

Strong candidates will also discuss the implications of the results, particularly regarding the use of alcohol dehydrogenase inhibitors and haemodialysis.

[54] Gee P and Martin M. Toxic cocktail: Methanol poisoning in a tourist to Indonesia. *EMA* 2012 24(4): 451 - 453

PROBLEM 27.

A 45 year old man attends your emergency department with dizziness, chest pain and dyspnoea after ingesting sildenafil tablets and amyl nitrate bulbs at a local spa facility.

His vital signs are:

HR	120	/min
BP	80/40	mmHg
RR	30	/min
Sats	80%	60% O_2
T	37.3	°C

Arterial blood gas analysis is shown below.

Describe and interpret the results (100%).

FiO_2	0.6		
pH	7.2		
pO_2	400	mmHg	(53.3 kPa)
pCO_2	32	mmHg	(4.3 kPa)
HCO_3^-	16	mmol/L	
BE	-6		
O_2 sats	100%		
Na^+	128	mmol/L	
K^+	6.2	mmol/L	
Cl^-	92	mmol/L	
Lactate	4.5	mmol/L	

ANSWER

1. Acid-Base Balance

Moderate acidaemia

Mild hypocapnoea
Respiratory alkalosis

Moderately low bicarbonate
Metabolic acidosis
Expect pCO2 = (8 + 1.5x16)
= 32mmHg
.: Dx appropriate compensation
Anion Gap
= 128 - (92+16)
= 128 - 108
= 20
Delta Ratio
= (20 - 12)/(24 - 16)
= 8/8
= 1.0
Therefore diagnose isolated RAGMA

Overall picture: RAGMA plus compensatory respiratory alkalosis

2. Oxygenation

A-a gradient FiO2 60%
= 450 - (1.25 x 32) - 400
= 450 - 40 - 400
= 450 - 440
= 10
Expect A-a grad for 45yo man = 45/4 + 4 = 15mmHg

Therefore non elevated A-a gradient suggests no V/Q mismatch exists.

3. Biochemistry

Mild hyponatraemia

Check BSL

Moderate hyperkalaemia

Expect K+ for pH 7.20 = 5 + (2 x 0.5) = 6.2 mmol/L

K+ level appropriate for pH

Significantly elevated lactate

Likely cause of RAGMA

Significant difference between measured sats and O2 sats probe

Saturation gap = 100 - 80 = 20%

4. Interpret

Critically ill man

Shocked

Tissue hypoxia

Primary disturbance is RAGMA due to lactate

Suggests tissue hypoxia in the context of arterial normoxia

Type A lactic acidosis

Other causes include

Type B1: sepsis/underlying disease (eg liver failure)

Type B2: drug OD, esp toxic alcohols

DDx

Methaemoglobinaemia given Hx nitrate use

Severe anaemia

Haemolysis, bleeding

Therefore check Hb and MetHb level

Inspect blood --> “chocolate coloured”

If MetHb elevated administer methylene blue 2mg/kg IV

A-a gradient in kPa

A-a gradient FiO_2 60%

= 60kPa – (1.25 x 4.3) – 53.3

= 60 – 5.3 – 53.3

= 60 – 58.6

= 1.4

Not Elevated (<2.5 kPa).

COMMENTS

A 45 year old man attends your emergency department with dizziness, chest pain and dyspnoea after ingesting sildenafil tablets and amyl nitrate bulbs at a local spa facility.

The mention of amyl nitrate in the stem provides a valuable clue to the answer for this interesting question. Astute candidates will also note the significant difference in oxygen saturations between the pulse oximetry value and the calculated value on the gas analyzer. The presence of methaemoglobin is associated with a falsely low reading on pulse oximetry[55], which is discrepant with the value calculated by the gas analyzer. (The gas analyzer is also incorrect, because the calculation assumes a normal O_2-Hb dissociation curve, which is not the case in these patients!)

Recreational use of amyl nitrate has been reported as a cause of methaemoglobinaemia[56], and this presentation should alert candidates to the need to evaluate for the presence of the pathology. Outstanding candidates will mention the visual inspection of blood and the use of methylene blue to display their knowledge of toxicology for maximum marks.

[55] Hamirani YS, Franklin W, Grifka RG and Stainback RF. Methemoglobinemia in a Young Man. *Tex Heart Inst J.* 2008; 35(1): 76 – 77

[56] Faley B and Chase H. A case of severe amyl nitrate induced methemoglobinemia managed with methylene blue. *J Clin Toxicol* 2012; 2:4

PROBLEM 28

A 70 year old woman attends your emergency department in severe respiratory distress. She has a history of COPD on home oxygen, as well as congestive cardiac failure and stage IV chronic kidney disease.

Her vital signs are:

HR	150	/min
BP	240/140mmHg	
RR	50	/min
Sats	68%	60% O_2
T	38.3	°C

Arterial blood gas analysis is shown below.

Describe and interpret the results. (100%).

FiO_2	0.6		
pH	7.2		
pO_2	45	mmHg	(6.0 kPa)
pCO_2	49	mmHg	(6.5 kPa)
HCO_3^-	19	mmol/L	
BE	-1		
Na^+	135	mmol/L	
K^+	5.4	mmol/L	
Cl^-	93	mmol/L	
Lactate	8.5	mmol/L	

ANSWER

1. Acid-Base Balance

Mild - Moderate acidaemia

Mild hypercapnoea

Respiratory acidosis

Expect HCO_3^- = 25 acutely or 28 chronically

Mild decrease bicarbonate

Metabolic acidosis

Expect pCO_2 = (8 + 1.5x19)

= 36.5mmHg

.: Dx combined metabolic and respiratory acidosis

Anion Gap

= 135 - (93+19)

= 135 - 112

= 23

Delta Ratio

= (23 - 12)/(24 - 19)

= 11/5

= >2.0

Therefore diagnose RAGMA plus pre-existing metabolic alkalosis

Note fall in HCO3- excessive for change in BE

Overall picture: triple disturbance as described

2. Oxygenation

A-a gradient for FiO_2 60%

= 450 - (1.25 x 49) - 45

= 450 - 61 - 45

= 450 - 106

= 344

Expect A-a grad for 70yo woman = 70/4 + 4 = ~22mmHg

Therefore Dx critically elevated A-a gradient and severe respiratory failure. Profound V/Q mismatch:

Likely combined pathology given history
APO (CCF)
Bronchopneumonia (COPD)
ARDS (SIRS/aspiration)
Interstitial lung disease
Other respiratory membrane disease
PE

3. Biochemistry

Normonatraemia
Mild hyperkalaemia
Expect K+ for pH 7.20 = 5 + (2 x 0.5) = 6.2 mmol/L
Therefore mild relative hypokalaemia, watch K+ as pH corrected
Mild hypochloraemia
Electrical equilibration RAGMA
Significantly elevated lactate
Likely cause of RAGMA

4. Interpret

Critically ill pt
Life threatening hypoxia despite supplemental O2
Severe exacerbation COPD/CCF
Likely chronic metabolic alkalosis secondary COPD (triple disturbance)
RAGMA - hyperlactataemia
A - profound hypoxia due to respiratory failure
B_1 - sepsis
B_2 - possible drug accumulation (eg renal failure + metformin toxicity)
Also check BSL (DKA) and renal indices RE acidosis

Meets indications for BiPAP
Resuscitate/treat for infective exacerbation COPD, APO (GTN infusion) and respiratory sepsis with broad spectrum Abx

A-a gradient in kPa

A-a gradient FiO_2 60%
= 60 kPa – (1.25 x 6.5) – 6.0
= 60 – 7.5 – 6.0
= 60 – 13.5
= 46.5

Grossly Elevated (>2.5 kPa).

COMMENTS

A 70 year old woman attends your emergency department in severe respiratory distress. She has a history of COPD on home oxygen, as well as congestive cardiac failure and stage IV chronic kidney disease.

Candidates with some emergency experience will be familiar with such complex and diagnostically challenging presentations. There is a broad range of potential differential diagnoses relating to multiple organ systems, and the key to answering this question is to work through the blood gas in a systematic fashion.

Addressing the initial blood gas disturbance, it is clear that the patient has a raised anion gap metabolic acidosis. However, candidates who are becoming astute at reading blood gases will no doubt notice a significant discrepancy between the fall in bicarbonate and the minor decrease in base excess, and realize that this implies the simultaneous presence of a metabolic alkalosis. Of course, many patients with COPD do indeed have a pre-extant alkalosis as a buffer for chronic CO2 retention. The application of the delta ratio to the anion gap clearly reveals that there is indeed a metabolic alkalosis underlying the acidosis, and with the presence of a respiratory alkalosis a triple disturbance can be diagnosed.

The key is working systematically, which has been the focus of this book.

For perspective candidates should mention that this patient is critically ill. The substantially elevated Aa gradient should be delineated, and strong answers will finish with a sensible statement as to where the clinician would like to proceed both diagnostically and therapeutically.

PROBLEM 29

A 50 year old farmer presents after taking an unknown overdose. He has pinpoint pupils, and is hyper salivating and flushed. The ambulance reports profound diarrhoea prior to his arrival in the ED.

His vital signs are:

HR	28	/min
BP	80/45	mmHg
RR	4	/min
Sats	70%	40% O_2
T	36.3	°C

Arterial blood gas analysis is shown below.

Describe and interpret the results. (100%).

FiO_2	0.4		
pH	6.85		
pO_2	125	mmHg	(16.7 kPa)
pCO_2	130	mmHg	(17.3 kPa)
HCO_3^-	10	mmol/L	
BE	-14		
Na^+	140	mmol/L	
K^+	4.5	mmol/L	
Cl^-	104	mmol/L	
Lactate	11	mmol/L	

ANSWER

1. Acid-Base Balance

Life threatening acidaemia

Significant hypercapnoea

Respiratory acidosis

Expect HCO_3^- = 27 acutely or 36 chronically

Severe decrease bicarbonate

Metabolic acidosis

Expect pCO_2 = (8 + 1.5x10)

= 23mmHg

.: Dx combined metabolic and respiratory acidosis

Anion Gap

= 140 - (104 + 10)

= 140 - 114

= 26

Delta Ratio

= (26 - 12)/(24 - 10)

= 14/14

= 1.0

Therefore diagnose isolated RAGMA.

Overall picture is a double disturbance: respiratory acidosis + RAGMA

2. Oxygenation

A-a gradient for FiO_2 40%

= 300 - (1.25 x 130) - 125

= 300 – 162.5 - 125

= 300 – 287.5

= 12.5

Expect A-a grad for 50yo man = 50/4 + 4 = ~16mmHg

Therefore Dx normal A-a gradient

respiratory failure due to isolated hypoventilation

3. Biochemistry

Normonatraemia
Normokalaemia
Expect K+ for pH 6.85 = 5 + (5.5 x 0.5) = 7.75 mmol/L
Therefore significant relative hypokalaemia, watch K+ as pH corrected
Normochloraemia
Critically elevated lactate
Likely cause of RAGMA

4. Interpret

Critically ill man
Overdose with symptoms of cholinergic poisoning
Bradycardic and haemodynamic compromise: atropine indicated
Suggests organophosphate poisoning
Causes of RAGMA
Hyperlactataemia
A - profound hypoxia
- due to respiratory failure prior to O2 administration
- hypoperfusion due to bradycardia and shock
B_1 - sepsis/aspiration
B_2 - possible drug accumulation, or other overdose

High dose atropine +/- pralidoxime indicated
PPI for staff RE risk of cross contamination

A-a gradient in kPa

A-a gradient FiO_2 40%
= 40 kPa – (1.25 x 17.3) – 16.7
= 40 – 21.6 – 16.7
= 40 – 38.3
= 1.7

Not Elevated (<2.5 kPa).

COMMENTS

A 50 year old farmer presents after taking an unknown overdose. He has pinpoint pupils, and is hyper salivating and flushed. The ambulance reports profound diarrhoea prior to his arrival in the ED.

The stem clearly points towards candidates towards a toxicological exposure for this presentation. Candidates with a basic knowledge of toxicology will recognize the symptoms of cholinergic overload which is a cardinal manifestation of organophosphate poisoning, chemicals which are often used as pesticides[57].

Organophosphates are associated with acute paralysis and respiratory insufficiency[58], and evidence of an acute respiratory acidosis and tissue hypoxia are found when working through the question. The normal Aa gradient implies that the issue is respiratory insufficiency rather than pulmonary pathology which is the acute problem and candidates should specifically comment on this to clearly demonstrate their understanding of the pathology at work.

Strong answers will include the need for high dose atropine and/or pralidoxime, and exceptional answers will mention the need for staff PPE due to the risk of secondary exposure.

[57] Rose KR. Organophosphate exposure in Australian agricultural workers : human exposure and risk assessment. PhD thesis, Queensland University of Technology. Retrieved 17 January 2015 from http://eprints.qut.edu.au/16345/.

[58] Singh S, Sharma N. Neurological syndromes following organophosphate poisoning. *Neurol India* 2000;48:308

PROBLEM 30

A 3 year old girl is brought in by ambulance from a children's party. She has a known peanut allergy, and has developed acute dyspnoea and stridor after eating a piece of birthday cake.

Her vital signs are:

HR	180	/min
BP	65/45	mmHg
RR	45	/min
Sats	88%	40% O_2
T	37.1	°C

On arrival to the emergency department she is cyanosed with stridor and swollen lips.

Urgent venous blood gas analysis is shown below.

Describe and interpret the results. (70%)

Outline your treatment priorities. (30%).

FiO_2	0.4		
pH	7.15		
pO_2	45	mmHg	(5.99 kPa)
pCO_2	60	mmHg	(7.99 kPa)
HCO_3^-	12	mmol/L	
BE	-12		
Na^+	138	mmol/L	
K^+	5.5	mmol/L	
Cl^-	102	mmol/L	
Lactate	5.5	mmol/L	

ANSWER

1. Acid-Base Balance

Severe acidaemia

Significant hypercapnoea

Respiratory acidosis

Expect HCO_3^- = 26 acutely or 32 chronically

Moderate decrease bicarbonate

Metabolic acidosis

Expect pCO_2 = (8 + 1.5x12)

= 26mmHg

.: Dx combined metabolic and respiratory acidosis

Anion Gap

= 138 - (102 + 12)

= 138 - 114

= 24

Delta Ratio

= (24 - 12)/(24 - 12)

= 12/12

= 1.0

Therefore diagnose isolated RAGMA.

Therefore diagnose dual disturbance: resp acidosis and RAGMA

2. Oxygenation

A-a n/a as VBG

Note significant hypoxia on supplemental O2 on clinical exam

3. Biochemistry

Normonatraemia

Mild hyperkalaemia

Expect K+ for pH 7.15 = 5 + (2.5 x 0.5) = 6.25 mmol/L

Therefore mild relative hypokalaemia, watch K+ as pH corrected

Normochloraemia

Significantly elevated lactate
Likely cause of RAGMA

4. Interpret

Critically ill child
Impending airway obstruction and hypotension secondary to anaphylaxis
Complicated by respiratory acidosis and RAGMA
RAGMA
Causes of RAGMA
Hyperlactataemia
A - profound hypoxia
airway obstruction and shock
B1 - sepsis/aspiration
B2 - overdose unlikely but clarify history
B3 - paediatric, possible inborn error of metabolism

TREATMENT PRIORITIES

3yo child
Estimate weight 16kg
ETT 4.0 tube

Resuscitate
Immediate access IV/IO
Fluid bolus NaCl 0.9% 20ml/kg repeat as necessary
High flow O2
Prepare to secure airway - RSI/Jet insufflation

Treat Anaphylaxis
Immediate IM adrenaline 10mcg/kg = 160mcg
IV hydrocortisone and non sedating antihistamine
Prepare adrenaline infusion

Manage parents
Information/delegate staff member

COMMENTS

A 3 year old girl is brought in by ambulance from a children's party. She has a known peanut allergy, and has developed acute dyspnoea and stridor after eating a piece of birthday cake.

On arrival to the emergency department she is cyanosed with stridor and swollen lips.

This stem clearly indicates a diagnosis of acute anaphylaxis, and candidates should proceed through the subsequent calculations without too much difficulty to find an acute respiratory acidosis combined with an acute metabolic acidosis.

To answer this question correctly at specialist level candidates need to recognize that this patient is in imminent danger of death. This should be clearly spelled out in the interpretation of the gas. It is even prompted for by a second question, asking for treatment priorities. As part of this the entire spectrum of paediatric resuscitation should be briefly covered, including an estimated weight and management of the parents as well as the paediatric patient. Candidates must include the administration of an appropriate weight based dose of IM adrenaline to pass this highly clinically focused question.

THE EXTENDED MATCH QUESTIONS

"You sort of start thinking anything's possible if you've got enough nerve."

J.K.Rowling.

How to approach an EMQ.

We have included this section for several reasons and we feel there is some value for everyone.

For those sitting the ACEM fellowship exam the EMQs provide an opportunity to practice for the biggest examination of your career. For colleagues sitting other exams which have an element of extended match or multiple choice these questions likewise provide an opportunity to test your knowledge.

Alternatively for those who have simply sought to improve their skills in interpreting the blood gas, each of the EMQs can be used as the first thirty questions in this book are. Answers are provided after each paper for you to check yourself.

We reiterate at this stage that you should approach these EMQs with our systematic approach. Ask yourself:

1. What is the major acid base disturbance?
2. What is the Aa gradient?
3. What are the relevant electrolyte disturbances?
4. What can I infer about diagnosis and management, especially with the clinical information I have to hand?

As always, a systematic approach is the key! Good luck.

EMQ PAPER 1.

For each clinical scenario provided:

1. Describe the major acid base balance disturbances and any compensatory response.
2. Calculate an anion gap and delta ratio where applicable.
3. Calculate an A-a gradient where applicable.
4. Perform any other calculations you consider relevant.
5. Select an appropriate diagnosis from the stems below.

1) *Acute pulmonary oedema*
2) *Ethanol toxicity*
3) *Anaphylaxis with impaired gas exchange*
4) *Brown snake (Pseudonaja spp) envenomation*
5) *Frusemide toxicity*
6) *Bicarbonate loss from the GIT*
7) *Pyloric stenosis*
8) *Seizure induced hyperlactataemia*
9) *Carbon monoxide toxicity*
10) *Isoniazid toxicity*
11) *Gastrointestinal perforation*
12) *Septic shock*
13) *Sodium valproate toxicity*
14) *Methanol toxicity*
15) *Cushing's syndrome*
16) *Cardiogenic shock*
17) *Hepatic encephalopathy*
18) *Tiger snake (Notechis spp) envenomation*
19) *Taipan (Oxyuranus spp) envenomation*
20) *Bicarbonate loss from the renal tract*
21) *Gastrointestinal perforation*
22) *Acute pancreatitis*
23) *Acute crush syndrome*
24) *Black snake (Pseudechis spp) envenomation*
25) *Diabetic ketoacidosis*
26) *Metformin toxicity*
27) *Major gastrointestinal haemorrhage*
28) *Ethylene glycol toxicity*
29) *Anaphylaxis with airway compromise*
30) *Acute adrenal insufficiency*
31) *Bowel obstruction*
32) *Cyanide toxicity*
33) *Death adder (Acanthopis) envenomation*
34) *Acetazolamide toxicity*
35) *Drug induced renal failure*
36) *Spironolactone toxicity*

QUESTION 1.1

A 36 year old male presents after being bitten by a snake.

His vital signs are:

HR	105	/min
BP	125/80	mmHg
RR	26	/min
Sats	100%	RA
T	37.2	°C

An arterial blood gas is taken.

FiO_2	0.21		
pH	7.10		
pO_2	100	mmHg	(13.3 kPa)
pCO_2	32	mmHg	(4.3 kPa)
HCO_3^-	16	mmol/L	
BE	-8		
Na^+	138	mmol/L	
K^+	5.5	mmol/L	
Cl^-	112	mmol/L	
Urea	10	mmol/L	
Creatinine	300	μmol/L	
Lactate	1.2	mmol/L	
INR	1.0		
CK	15,000	IU/L	

QUESTION 1.2

A 25 year old epileptic presents with a an acute confusional state.

His vital signs are:

HR	111	/min
BP	121/87 mmHg	
RR	18	/min
Sats	100%	40% O_2
T	37.8	°C

An arterial blood gas is taken.

FiO_2	0.4		
pH	6.95		
pO_2	205	mmHg	(27.3 kPa)
pCO_2	60	mmHg	(8.0 kPa)
HCO_3^-	16	mmol/L	
BE	-8		
Lactate	7.0	mmol/L	
Na^+	152	mmol/L	
K^+	7.0	mmol/L	
Cl^-	114	mmol/L	
Urea	7.2	mmol/L	
Creatinine	83	μmol/L	

QUESTION 1.3.

A 73 year old man with a history of atrial fibrillation presents with severe sudden onset central abdominal pain. He has no acute surgical signs on examination, but does have an acutely tender abdomen.

His vital signs are:

HR	121	/min
BP	137/98 mmHg	
RR	36	/min
Sats	100%	RA
T	37.1	°C

An arterial blood gas is taken.

FiO_2	0.21		
pH	7.12		
pO_2	103	mmHg	(13.7 kPa)
pCO_2	26	mmHg	(3.5 kPa)
HCO_3^-	12	mmol/L	
BE	-10		
Na^+	147	mmol/L	
K^+	4.6	mmol/L	
Cl^-	110	mmol/L	
Urea	9.8	mmol/L	
Creatinine	105	μmol/L	
Lactate	4.9	mmol/L	

QUESTION 1.4

A 4 year old boy has developed acute stridor after being stung by a bee.

His vital signs are:

HR	145	/min
BP	78/56	mmHg
RR	38	/min
Sats	100%	28% O_2
T	36.8	°C

An arterial blood gas is taken.

FiO_2	0.28		
pH	7.12		
pO_2	98	mmHg	(13.1 kPa)
pCO_2	75	mmHg	(10.0 kPa)
HCO_3^-	19	mmol/L	
Na^+	142	mmol/L	
K^+	5.5	mmol/L	
Cl^-	106	mmol/L	
Urea	6.5	mmol/L	
Creatinine	54	µmol/L	
Lactate	4.1	mmol/L	

QUESTION 1.5

A 19 year old female presents after overdosing on her anti-epileptic medication.

Her vital signs are:

HR	118	/min
BP	80/58	mmHg
RR	24	/min
Sats	100%	RA
T	37.1	°C

An arterial blood gas is taken.

FiO_2	0.21		
pH	7.15		
pO_2	104	mmHg	(13.9 kPa)
pCO_2	32	mmHg	(4.26 kPa)
HCO_3^-	16	mmol/L	
BE	-8		
Na^+	139	mmol/L	
K^+	5.8	mmol/L	
Cl^-	104	mmol/L	
Urea	4.2	mmol/L	
Creatinine	67	µmol/L	
Ammonium	160	umol/L	
Lactate	5.2mmol/L		

QUESTION 1.6

A 35 year old female with a history of Crohn's disease and ileostomy presents with high volume output from her stoma.

Her vital signs are:

HR	123	/min
BP	103/86 mmHg	
RR	30	/min
Sats	100%	RA
T	38.1	°C

An arterial blood gas is taken.

FiO_2	0.21		
pH	7.14		
pO_2	107	mmHg	(14.3 kPa)
pCO_2	29	mmHg	(3.9 kPa)
HCO_3^-	14	mmol/L	
BE	-6		
Lactate	0.8	mmol/L	
Na^+	142	mmol/L	
K^+	5.1	mmol/L	
Cl^-	114	mmol/L	
Urea	8.9	mmol/L	
Creatinine	99	µmol/L	

QUESTION 1.7

A 65 year old man with a history of ischaemic heart disease presents at 6am with acute dyspnoea and a cough productive of pink frothy sputum.

His vital signs are:

HR	144	/min
BP	187/64 mmHg	
RR	29	/min
Sats	93%	60% O_2
T	37.0	°C

An arterial blood gas is taken.

FiO_2	0.6		
pH	7.13		
pO_2	78	mmHg	(10.4 kPa)
pCO_2	55	mmHg	(7.3 kPa)
HCO_3^-	26	mmol/L	
BE	+2		
Na^+	135	mmol/L	
K^+	5.3	mmol/L	
Cl^-	104	mmol/L	
Urea	5.7	mmol/L	
Creatinine	93	μmol/L	
Lactate	2.3mmol/L		

QUESTION 1.8

A four year old boy presents with a fever and purpuric rash. He has a decreased level of consciousness and poor respiratory effort.

His vital signs are:

HR	165	/min
BP	72/41	mmHg
RR	41	/min
Sats	100%	60% O_2
T	39.9	°C

An arterial blood gas is taken.

FiO_2	0.60		
pH	6.72		
PO_2	109	mmHg	(14.5 kPa)
PCO_2	65	mmHg	(8.7 kPa)
HCO_3	8.6	mmol/L	
BE	-16		
Na^+	140	mmol/L	
K^+	6.2	mmol/L	
Cl^-	104	mmol/L	
Urea	19.2	mmol/L	
Creatinine	200	μmol/L	
Lactate	10.1	mmol/L	

QUESTION 1.9

A 16 year old girl presents with poorly localized chest pain and dyspnoea. She is teary and distressed by the pain.

Her vital signs are:

HR	105	/min
BP	119/81 mmHg	
RR	40	/min
Sats	100%	RA
T	37.0	°C

An arterial gas is taken.

FiO_2	0.21		
pH	7.61		
pO_2	122	mmHg	(16.3 kPa)
pCO_2	22	mmHg	(2.9 kPa)
HCO_3^-	20	mmol/L	
BE	-4		
Na+	139	mmol/L	
K+	4.0	mmol/L	
Cl-	111	mmol/L	
Urea	4.5	mmol/L	
Creatinine	80	µmol/L	
Lactate	1.1mmol/L		

QUESTION 1.10

A 45 year old man presents with acute visual loss after drinking homemade spirits.

His vital signs are:

HR	113	/min
BP	101/76 mmHg	
RR	34	/min
Sats	100%	RA
T	37.3	°C

An arterial blood gas is taken.

FiO_2	0.21		
pH	7.1		
pO_2	99	mmHg	(13.0 kPa)
pCO_2	17	mmHg	(2.3 kPa)
HCO_3^-	8	mmol/L	
BE	-18		
Na^+	149	mmol/L	
K^+	6.1	mmol/L	
Cl^-	115	mmol/L	
Urea	6.7	mmol/L	
Creatinine	80	µmol/L	
Lactate	7.8	mmol/L	
Glucose	8.5	mmol/L	
Osm_m	350	mosm/kg	

EMQ 1 ANSWERS

QUESTION 1.1

1. **Acid base disturbance**
   Primary metabolic acidosis and compensatory respiratory alkalosis (expected CO_2 32 mmHg).
2. **Anion Gap (AG) and Delta Ratio**
   AG 10.
   DR not applicable in this instance.
3. **A-a gradient in mmHg (kPa)**
   10mmHg (2.32 kPa)
4. **Other relevant calculations**
   U:C ratio 0.3
5. **Diagnosis.**
   Black snake envenomation.

Comment: *a major feature of envenomation with snakes of the genus Pseudechis is rhabdomyolysis in the absence of coagulopathy or respiratory failure. The low urea to creatinine ratio implies renal failure secondary to a high CK titre.*

QUESTION 1.2

1. **Acid base disturbance**
   Combined primary metabolic acidosis and primary respiratory acidosis.
2. **Anion Gap (AG) and Delta Ratio**
   AG 22
   DR 1.25
3. **A-a gradient in mmHg (kPa)**
   10mmHg (1.34 kPa)
4. **Other relevant calculations**
   Nil applicable
5. **Diagnosis.**
   Seizure induced hyperlactataemia.

Comment: *This patient has most likely had a seizure with a type A lactic acidosis caused by increased tissue oxygen demand, and an acute hypoventilation syndrome from respiratory muscle dysfunction associated with the seizure.*

QUESTION 1.3

1. **Acid base disturbance**

   Primary metabolic out acidosis with a compensatory metabolic alkalosis (expected CO_2 26mmHg)
2. **Anion Gap (AG) and Delta Ratio**

   AG 25.

   DR 1.08
3. **A-a gradient in mmHg (kPa)**

   14.5mmHg (2.95 kPa)
4. **Other relevant calculations**

   Nil applicable
5. **Diagnosis.**

   Mesenteric Ischaemia

Comment: *sudden onset abdominal pain and a raised lactate in a patient with risk factors for arterial thromboembolism raises the specter of mesenteric ischaemia.*

QUESTION 1.4

1. **Acid base disturbance**

   Combined metabolic acidosis and respiratory acidosis.
2. **Anion Gap (AG) and Delta Ratio**

   AG 17.

   DR 1.0
3. **A-a gradient in mmHg (kPa)**

   8.25mmHg (2.4 kPa)
4. **Other relevant calculations**

   Nil applicable
5. **Diagnosis.**

   Anaphylaxis with acute airway compromise.

Comment: *the given history clearly implies anaphylaxis, and the presence of hypercapnoea without elevation of the A-a gradient suggests an acute airway instruction with resultant hypoventilation.*

QUESTION 1.5

1. **Acid base disturbance**
   Metabolic acidosis with compensatory respiratory acidosis (expect CO_2 32mmHg)
2. **Anion Gap (AG) and Delta Ratio**
   AG 19
   DR 0.875
3. **A-a gradient in mmHg (kPa)**
   6mmHg (1.77 kPa)
4. **Other relevant calculations**
   Nil applicable
5. **Diagnosis.**
   Sodium valproate toxicity.

Comment: *Valproic acid impairs the initiation of the urea cycle at the mitochondrial level and is associated with a lactic acidosis and a high serum ammonium level.*

QUESTION 1.6

1. **Acid base disturbance**
   Metabolic acidosis and compensatory respiratory alkalosis (expect CO_2 29mmHg)
2. **Anion Gap (AG) and Delta Ratio**
   AG 14
   DR 0.2
3. **A-a gradient in mmHg (kPa)**
   6.75mmHg (1.82 kPa)
4. **Other relevant calculations**
   Urea:Creatinine ratio 89.8
5. **Diagnosis.**
   Bicarbonate loss from the GIT

Comment: *Working through the question clearly indicates a non anion gap acidosis, and in conjunction with the information in the stem excessive* *stomal loss of bicarbonate rich fluid can be inferred. Excess fluid loss also appears to have created an element of pre-renal failure, judging by the elevated urea:creatinine ratio.*

QUESTION 1.7

1. **Acid base disturbance**
   Respiratory acidosis and compensatory metabolic alkalosis (expect HCO_3^- 25 acutely and 28 chronically)
2. **Anion Gap (AG) and Delta Ratio**
   AG not applicable (alkalosis)
   DR not applicable (alkalosis)
3. **A-a gradient in mmHg (kPa)**
   303mmHg (40.43 kPa)
4. **Other relevant calculations**
   Nil applicable
5. **Diagnosis.**
   Acute pulmonary oedema

Comment: *This is a classic presentation to the emergency department as anyone who has worked a night shift will know! The gas results indicate a V/Q mismatch complicated by hypercapnoea and the history clearly suggests acute pulmonary oedema. This question again highlights the importance of always using all the information given in an exam.*

QUESTION 1.8

1. **Acid base disturbance**
   Combined primary metabolic acidosis and respiratory acidosis
2. **Anion Gap (AG) and Delta Ratio**
   AG 27
   DR 0.97
3. **A-a gradient in mmHg (kPa)**
   259mmHg (34.6 kPa)
4. **Other relevant calculations**
   Urea:creatinine ratio 96
5. **Diagnosis.**
   Septic shock

Comment: *The combination of profound raised anion gap metabolic acidosis, hyperlactataemia, respiratory insufficiency with a V/Q mismatch and elevated A-a gradient all suggest septic shock complicated by multiple organ dysfunction.*

QUESTION 1.9

1. **Acid base disturbance**

   Primary respiratory alkalosis with compensatory metabolic acidosis (expect HCO_3^- acutely 20 and chronically 14 chronically)
2. **Anion Gap (AG) and Delta Ratio**

   AG not applicable (alkalosis)

   DR not applicable (alkalosis)
3. **A-a gradient in mmHg (kPa)**

   0.5mmHg (<1 kPa)
4. **Other relevant calculations**

   Nil applicable
5. **Diagnosis.**

   Acute anxiety disorder

Comment: *An isolated respiratory alkalosis accompanied by a normal Aa gradient is typical of an acute anxiety attack.*

QUESTION 1.10

1. **Acid base disturbance**

   Metabolic acidosis and compensatory respiratory acidosis (expect CO_2 20mmHg)
2. **Anion Gap (AG) and Delta Ratio**

   AG 26

   DR 0.875
3. **A-a gradient in mmHg (kPa)**

   30mmHg (5.1 kPa)
4. **Other relevant calculations**

   Osm_c 313 mosm/kg

   Osm gap 37 mosm/kg
5. **Diagnosis.**

   Methanol toxicity

Comment: *Together with the raised anion gap metabolic acidosis the osmolar gap implies toxic alcohol ingestion. The normal renal function combined with visual loss suggests methanol intoxication.*

EMQ PAPER 2.

For each clinical scenario provided:

1. Describe the major acid base balance disturbances and any compensatory response.
2. Calculate an anion gap and delta ratio where applicable.
3. Calculate an A-a gradient where applicable.
4. Perform any other calculations you consider relevant.
5. Select an appropriate diagnosis from the stems below.

1) Acute pulmonary oedema
2) Ethanol toxicity
3) Anaphylaxis with impaired gas exchange
4) Brown snake (Pseudonaja spp) envenomation
5) Frusemide toxicity
6) Bicarbonate loss from the GIT
7) Pyloric stenosis
8) Seizure induced hyperlactataemia
9) Carbon monoxide toxicity
10) Isoniazid toxicity
11) Gastrointestinal perforation
12) Septic shock
13) Sodium valproate toxicity
14) Methanol toxicity
15) Cushing's syndrome
16) Cardiogenic shock
17) Hepatic encephalopathy
18) Tiger snake (Notechis spp) envenomation
19) Taipan (Oxyuranus spp) envenomation
20) Bicarbonate loss from the renal tract
21) Gastrointestinal perforation
22) Acute pancreatitis
23) Acute crush syndrome
24) Black snake (Pseudechis spp) envenomation
25) Diabetic ketoacidosis
26) Metformin toxicity
27) Major gastrointestinal haemorrhage
28) Ethylene glycol toxicity
29) Anaphylaxis with airway compromise
30) Acute adrenal insufficiency
31) Bowel obstruction
32) Cyanide toxicity
33) Death adder (Acanthopis) envenomation
34) Acetazolamide toxicity
35) Drug induced renal failure
36) Spironolactone toxicity

QUESTION 2.1

A 59 year old female with a history of cirrhosis presents with an altered level of consciousness.

Her vital signs are:

HR	89	/min
BP	162/85	mmHg
RR	10	/min
Sats	100%	RA
T	36.5	°C

An arterial blood gas is taken.

FiO_2	0.21		
pH	7.20		
pO_2	92	mmHg	(12.3 kPa)
pCO_2	48	mmHg	(6.4 kPa)
HCO_3^-	18	mmol/L	
BE	-6		
Na^+	139	mmol/L	
K^+	7.0	mmol/L	
Cl^-	104	mmol/L	
Urea	2.2	mmol/L	
Creatinine	45	μmol/L	
Lactate	3.4	mmol/L	
Ammonium	84	μmol/L	

QUESTION 2.2

A 21 year old is retrieved by the trauma helicopter after a prolonged entrapment in a building collapse.

His vital signs are:

HR	119	/min
BP	97/62	mmHg
RR	36	/min
Sats	100%	40% O_2
T	37.1	°C

An arterial blood gas is taken.

FiO_2	0.4		
pH	7.02		
pO_2	126	mmHg	(16.8 kPa)
pCO_2	65	mmHg	(8.7 kPa)
HCO_3^-	13	mmol/L	
BE	-10		
Na^+	140	mmol/L	
K^+	8.2	mmol/L	
Cl^-	107	mmol/L	
Urea	7.7	mmol/L	
Creatinine	87	µmol/L	
Lactate	7.8	mmol/L	
CK	15000	IU/L	

QUESTION 2.3

An 86 year old woman with a history of congestive cardiac failure presents feeling unsteady on her feet.

HR	78	/min
BP	133/99	mmHg
RR	10	/min
Sats	100%	RA
T	36.6	°C

An arterial blood gas is taken.

FiO_2	0.21		
pH	7.65		
pO_2	88	mmHg	(11.7 kPa)
pCO_2	50	mmHg	(6.7 kPa)
HCO_3^-	36	mmol/L	
BE	+12		
Na^+	138	mmol/L	
K^+	2.2	mmol/L	
Cl^-	104	mmol/L	
Urea	13.2	mmol/L	
Creatinine	146	µmol/L	
Lactate	0.8	mmol/L	

QUESTION 2.4

A 9 year old boy presents with acute dyspnoea and dehydration.

His vital signs are:

HR	110	/min
BP	98/73	mmHg
RR	32	/min
Sats	100%	28% O_2
T	37.2	°C

An arterial blood gas is taken.

FiO_2	0.28		
pH	7.14		
PCO_2	26	mmHg	(3.5 kPa)
PO_2	158	mmHg	(21.0 kPa)
HCO_3	16	mmol/L	
Na^+	138	mmol/L	
K^+	6.23	mmol/L	
Cl^-	105	mmol/L	
Urea	9.7	mmol/L	
Creatinine	110	μmol/L	
Lactate	1.8	mmol/L	
Glucose	14.7	mmol/L	

QUESTION 2.5

A 25 year old presents after drinking anti-freeze solution.

Her vital signs are:

HR	111	/min
BP	105/70	mmHg
RR	29	/min
Sats	99%	RA
T	37.1	°C

An arterial blood gas is taken.

FiO_2	0.21		
pH	7.23		
pO_2	98	mmHg	(13.0 kPa)
pCO_2	24	mmHg	(3.2 kPa)
HCO_3^-	10	mmol/L	
BE	-14		
Na^+	136	mmol/L	
K^+	5.1	mmol/L	
Cl^-	96	mmol/L	
Urea	14	mmol/L	
Creatinine	240	µmol/L	
Lactate	6.2	mmol/L	
Glucose	6.4	mmol/L	
Osmolality	32	mosm/kg	

QUESTION 2.6

A 4 week old baby girl presents with projectile vomiting. (pyloric stenosis)

Her vital signs are:

HR	178	/min
BP	68/39	mmHg
RR	26	/min
Sats	100%	RA
T	36.7	°C

An arterial blood gas is taken.

FiO_2	0.21		
pH	7.55		
PO_2	99	mmHg	(13.2 kPa)
PCO_2	50	mmHg	(6.7 kPa)
HCO_3	28	mmol/L	
BE	+4		
Na^+	143	mmol/L	
K^+	3.8	mmol/L	
Cl^-	70	mmol/L	
Urea	2.1	mmol/L	
Creatinine	43	µmol/L	
Lactate	1.26	mmol/L	

QUESTION 2.7

A 62 year old woman with a history of bowel resection and end ileostomy formation presents with abdominal distention and copious vomiting. (dx acute bowel obstruction)

Her vital signs are:

HR	109	/min
BP	102/68	mmHg
RR	31	/min
Sats	100%	RA
T	37.1	°C

An arterial blood gas is taken.

FiO_2	0.21		
pH	7.58		
pO_2	98	mmHg	(13.0 kPa)
pCO_2	54	mmHg	(7.2 kPa)
HCO_3^-	28	mmol/L	
BE	+4		
Na^+	142	mmol/L	
K^+	3.2	mmol/L	
Cl^-	96	mmol/L	
Urea	10.2	mmol/L	
Creatinine	103	µmol/L	
Lactate	1.2	mmol/L	

QUESTION 2.8

A 60 year old female is referred from a migrant health centre after taking an overdose of an unknown antimicrobial agent.

Her vital signs are:

HR	123	/min
BP	87/68	mmHg
RR	26	/min
Sats	100%	RA
T	37.4	°C

An arterial blood gas is taken.

FiO_2	0.21		
pH	7.05		
pO_2	98	mmHg	(13.0 kPa)
pCO_2	35	mmHg	(4.7 kPa)
HCO_3^-	18	mmol/L	
BE	-6		
Na^+	142	mmol/L	
K^+	6.5	mmol/L	
Cl^-	104	mmol/L	
Urea	5.2	mmol/L	
Creatinine	89	μmol/L	
Lactate	7.2	mmol/L	
ALT	500	IU/L	
AST	650	IU/L	
GGT	86	IU/L	
ALP	106	IU/L	

QUESTION 2.9

A 45 year old woman presents with a two week history of profuse watery diarrhoea.

Her vital signs are:

HR	108	/min
BP	114/74	mmHg
RR	11	/min
Sats	100%	RA
T	37.9	°C

An arterial blood gas is taken.

FiO_2	0.21		
pH	7.26		
pO_2	106	mmHg	(14.1 kPa)
pCO_2	38	mmHg	(5.1 kPa)
HCO_3^-	20	mmol/L	
BE	-4		
Na^+	135	mmol/L	
K^+	5.6	mmol/L	
Cl^-	114	mmol/L	
Urea	21	mmol/L	
Creatinine	205	µmol/L	
Lactate	1.1	mmol/L	

QUESTION 2.10

A 84 year old woman presents with acute onset upper abdominal pain and malaena.

Her vital signs are:

HR	122	/min
BP	108/85	mmHg
RR	29	/min
Sats	100%	28% O_2
T	37.8	°C

An arterial blood gas is taken.

FiO_2	0.28		
pH	7.12		
PCO_2	32	mmHg	(4.26 kPa)
PO_2	145	mmHg	(19.3 kPa)
HCO_3^-	16	mmol/L	
BE	-8		
Na^+	142	mmol/L	
K^+	6.7	mmol/L	
Cl^-	106	mmol/L	
Urea	6.1	mmol/L	
Creatinine	86	µmol/L	
Lactate	5.75	mmol/L	

EMQ 2 ANSWERS

QUESTION 2.1

1. **Acid base disturbance**
   Combined metabolic acidosis and respiratory acidosis
2. **Anion Gap (AG) and Delta Ratio**
   AG 17
   DR 0.83
3. **A-a gradient in mmHg (kPa)**
   0mmHg (0 kPa)
4. **Other relevant calculations**
   Nil applicable
5. **Diagnosis.**
   Hepatic encephalopathy

Comment: *This patient with a given history of liver failure has an accumulation of lactate and ammonium with resultant hepatic encephalopathy and acute hypoventilation.*

QUESTION 2.2

1. **Acid base disturbance**
   Combined metabolic acidosis and respiratory acidosis
2. **Anion Gap (AG) and Delta Ratio**
   AG 20
   DR 0.7
3. **A-a gradient in mmHg (kPa)**
   92mmHg (12.3 kPa)
4. **Other relevant calculations**
   Urea:creatinine ratio 41
   Expect K^+ for pH to be 6.5mmol/L
5. **Diagnosis.**
   Acute crush syndrome

Comment: *This blood gas shows the acute sequelae of prolonged entrapment: rhabdomyolysis, hyperkalaemia (above that expected for the accompanying pH) and renal failure with a low urea:creatinine ratio. The associated hypoventilation and elevated V/Q mismatch likely represent significant pulmonary injury.*

QUESTION 2.3

1. **Acid base disturbance**
   Metabolic alkalosis with compensatory respiratory acidosis
2. **Anion Gap (AG) and Delta Ratio**
   AG not applicable (alkalosis)
   DR not applicable (alkalosis)
3. **A-a gradient in mmHg (kPa)**
   0mmHg (0 kPa)
4. **Other relevant calculations**
   Nil applicable
5. **Diagnosis.**
   Frusemide toxicity

Comment: *Frusemide, a drug commonly used for congestive cardiac failure is associated with hypokalaemia and metabolic alkalosis because of changes in electrolyte absorption in the renal tubules.*

QUESTION 2.4

1. **Acid base disturbance**
   Metabolic acidosis with compensatory respiratory alkalosis (expect CO_2 32mmHg)
2. **Anion Gap (AG) and Delta Ratio**
   AG 21
   DR 1.12
3. **A-a gradient in mmHg (kPa)**
   9.5mmHg (2.62 kPa)
4. **Other relevant calculations**
   Nil applicable
5. **Diagnosis.**
   Diabetic ketoacidosis

Comment: *This is a fairly typical clinical and biochemical presentation of new onset type 1 diabetes.*

QUESTION 2.5

1. **Acid base disturbance**

Metabolic acidosis and compensatory respiratory alkalosis

2. **Anion Gap (AG) and Delta Ratio**

   AG 30

   DR 1.28
3. **A-a gradient in mmHg (kPa)**

   22mmHg (4 kPa)
4. **Other relevant calculations**

   Urea:Creatinine ratio 58

   Osmc 296 mosm/kg

   Osmolar gap 34 mosm/Kg
5. **Diagnosis.**

   Ethylene glycol toxicity.

Comment: *Both methanol and ethylene glycol are associated with a raised osmolar gap and raised anion gap (lactic) acidosis. Ethylene glycol is metabolized to oxalate which precipitates in urine and may cause acute renal dysfunction.*

QUESTION 2.6

1. **Acid base disturbance**

   Metabolic alkalosis with compensatory respiratory acidosis.
2. **Anion Gap (AG) and Delta Ratio**

   AG not applicable (alkalosis)

   DR not applicable (alkalosis)
3. **A-a gradient in mmHg (kPa)**

   0mmHg (0 kPa)
4. **Other relevant calculations**

   Nil applicable
5. **Diagnosis.**

   Pyloric stenosis

Comment: *This is a classic presentation for pyloric stenosis, with the metabolic alkalosis and profound hypochloraemia caused by significant HCl loss with repeated vomiting.*

QUESTION 2.7

1. **Acid base disturbance**

   Metabolic alkalosis with compensatory respiratory acidosis.

2. Anion Gap (AG) and Delta Ratio

AG not applicable (alkalosis)

DR not applicable (alkalosis)

3. A-a gradient in mmHg (kPa)

0mmHg (0 kPa)

4. Other relevant calculations

Nil applicable

5. Diagnosis.

Bowel obstruction.

Comment: *The given history suggests a bowel obstruction, which produces a similar biochemical picture to pyloric stenosis.*

QUESTION 2.8

1. Acid base disturbance

Metabolic acidosis and compensatory respiratory alkalosis (expect CO_2 35mmHg)

2. Anion Gap (AG) and Delta Ratio

AG 20

DR 1.3

3. A-a gradient in mmHg (kPa)

8.25 mmHg (2.1 kPa)

4. Other relevant calculations

Nil applicable

5. Diagnosis.

Isoniazid toxicity

Comment: *Isoniazid toxicity is associated with hyperlactataemia and liver dysfunction, as well as agranulocytosis. It is a common drug used to treat tuberculosis and should be considered as a potential overdose in appropriate populations.*

QUESTION 2.9

1. Acid base disturbance

Metabolic acidosis.

2. Anion Gap (AG) and Delta Ratio

AG 1

DR not applicable (AG <12)

3. **A-a gradient in mmHg (kPa)**
   0 mmHg (0 kPa)
4. **Other relevant calculations**
   Urea:creatinine ratio 102
5. **Diagnosis.**
   Bicarbonate loss from the GIT

Comment: *Excessive loss of bicarbonate in bowel secretions is associated with a non anion gap metabolic acidosis.*

QUESTION 2.10

1. **Acid base disturbance**
   Metabolic aciosis and compensatory respiratory alkalosis.
2. **Anion Gap (AG) and Delta Ratio**
   AG 20
   DR 1.0
3. **A-a gradient in mmHg (kPa)**
   15mmHg (3.37 kPa)
4. **Other relevant calculations**
   Nil applicable
5. **Diagnosis.**
   Major gastrointestinal haemorrhage.

Comment: *This patient has clear evidence of haemodynamic instability and a history suggestive of upper GI bleed. It is likely that significant hypoperfusion has lead to the development of a type A lactic acidosis.*

EMQ PAPER 3.

For each clinical scenario provided:

1. Describe the major acid base balance disturbances and any compensatory response.
2. Calculate an anion gap and delta ratio where applicable.
3. Calculate an A-a gradient where applicable.
4. Perform any other calculations you consider relevant.
5. Select an appropriate diagnosis from the stems below.

(i) Acute pulmonary oedema
(ii) Ethanol toxicity
(iii) Anaphylaxis with impaired gas exchange
(iv) Brown snake (Pseudonaja spp) envenomation
(v) Frusemide toxicity
(vi) Bicarbonate loss from the GIT
(vii) Pyloric stenosis
(viii) Seizure induced hyperlactataemia
(ix) Carbon monoxide toxicity
(x) Isoniazid toxicity
(xi) Gastrointestinal perforation
(xii) Septic shock
(xiii) Sodium valproate toxicity
(xiv) Methanol toxicity
(xv) Cushing's syndrome
(xvi) Cardiogenic shock
(xvii) Hepatic encephalopathy
(xviii) Tiger snake (Notechis spp) envenomation
(xix) Taipan (Oxyuranus spp) envenomation
(xx) Bicarbonate loss from the renal tract
(xxi) Gastrointestinal perforation
(xxii) Acute pancreatitis
(xxiii) Acute crush syndrome
(xxiv) Black snake (Pseudechis spp) envenomation
(xxv) Diabetic ketoacidosis
(xxvi) Metformin toxicity
(xxvii) Major gastrointestinal haemorrhage
(xxviii) Ethylene glycol toxicity
(xxix)Anaphylaxis with airway compromise
(xxx) Acute adrenal insufficiency
(xxxi) Bowel obstruction
(xxxii) Cyanide toxicity
(xxxiii) Death adder (Acanthopis) envenomation
(xxxiv) Acetazolamide toxicity
(xxxv) Drug induced renal failure
(xxxvi) Spironolactone toxicity

QUESTION 3.1

A 16 year old male presents after being bitten by a snake.

His vital signs are:

HR	98	/min
BP	117/78	mmHg
RR	4	/min
Sats	100%	28% O_2
T	37.1	°C

An arterial blood gas is taken.

FiO_2	0.28		
pH	7.20		
pO_2	114	mmHg	(15.2 kPa)
pCO_2	70	mmHg	(9.3 kPa)
HCO_3^-	27	mmol/L	
BE	+4		
Na^+	140	mmol/L	
K^+	5.5	mmol/L	
Cl^-	107	mmol/L	
Urea	7	mmol/L	
Creatinine	86	μmol/L	
Lactate	1.2	mmol/L	
INR	1.0		
CK	67	IU/L	

QUESTION 3.2

An 84 year old man treated with frusemide for CCF and indomethacin for a lower back injury presents feeling dyspnoeic. He has a history of hypertension treated with an ACE inhibitor.

His vital signs are:

HR	115	/min
BP	146/98 mmHg	
RR	27	/min
Sats	100%	RA
T	37.1	°C

An arterial blood gas is taken.

FiO_2	0.21		
pH	7.10		
pO_2	107	mmHg	(14.3 kPa)
pCO_2	27	mmHg	(3.6 kPa)
HCO_3^-	13	mmol/L	
BE	-10		
Na^+	137	mmol/L	
K^+	5.0	mmol/L	
Cl^-	106	mmol/L	
urea	24	mmol/L	
creatinine	460	μmol/L	
Lactate	0.9	mmol/L	

QUESTION 3.3

An 11 year old boy presents with his mother with acute dyspnoea.

His vital signs are:

HR	152	/min
BP	99/72	mmHg
RR	45	/min
Sats	100%	40% O_2
T	37.7	°C

An arterial gas is taken.

FiO_2	0.40		
pH	6.92		
PO_2	260	mmHg	(34.7 kPa)
PCO_2	13	mmHg	(1.7 kPa)
HCO_3^-	3.1	mmol/L	
BE	-21		
Na^+	143	mmol/L	
K^+	2.2	mmol/L	
Cl^-	107	mmol/L	
Urea	6.2	mmol/L	
Creatinine	78	μmol/L	
Lactate	2.48	mmol/L	
Glucose	31.6	mmol/L	

QUESTION 3.4

A 27 year old woman presents with acute onset upper abdominal pain. She has a history of NSAID use for period pain, and her abdomen is peritonitic when examined.

Her vital signs are:

HR	114	/min
BP	110/82 mmHg	
RR	27	/min
Sats	100%	RA
T	38.2	°C

An arterial blood gas is taken.

FiO_2	0.21		
pH	7.14		
PCO_2	29	mmHg	(3.9 kPa)
PO_2	105	mmHg	(14.0 kPa)
HCO_3^-	14	mmol/L	
BE	-7		
Na^+	145	mmol/L	
K^+	6.2	mmol/L	
Cl^-	126	mmol/L	
Urea	16.2	mmol/L	
Creatinine	150	µmol/L	
Lactate	4.26mmol/L		

QUESTION 3.5

A 2 week old baby presents with a decreased level of consciousness after a seizure.

Her vital signs are:

HR	164	/min
BP	80/40	mmHg
RR	22	/min
Sats	100%	28% O_2
T	36.9	°C

A venous blood gas is taken.

FiO_2	0.28		
pH	7.07		
PCO_2	55	mmHg	(7.3 kPa)
PO_2	90	mmHg	(12.0 kPa)
HCO_3^-	17	mmol/L	
BE	-7		
Na^+	115	mmol/L	
K^+	7.1	mmol/L	
Cl^-	90	mmol/L	
Urea	3.1	mmol/L	
Creatinine	62	µmol/L	
Lactate	6.26	mmol/L	

QUESTION 3.6

A 70 year old male presents with an inferior infarct.

His vital signs are:

HR	111	/min	
BP	77/58	mmHg	
RR	34	/min	
Sats	100%	40% O_2	6L facemask
T	37.1	°C	

An arterial blood gas is taken.

FiO_2	0.40		
pH	7.27		
pO_2	152	mmHg	(20.3 kPa)
pCO_2	35	mmHg	(4.7 kPa)
HCO_3^-	19	mmol/L	
BE	-5		
Na^+	141	mmol/L	
K^+	4.6	mmol/L	
Cl^-	107	mmol/L	
Urea	17	mmol/L	
Creatinine	150	µmol/L	
Lactate	4.5	mmol/L	

QUESTION 3.7

A 4 year old boy presents after ingesting several of his grandmother's "fluid tablets".

His vital signs are:

HR	136	/min
BP	62/48	mmHg
RR	32	/min
Sats	100%	RA
T	36.9	°C

An arterial blood gas is taken.

FiO_2	0.21		
pH	7.25		
pO_2	102	mmHg	(13.6 kPa)
pCO_2	29	mmHg	(3.9 kPa)
HCO_3^-	14	mmol/L	
BE	-8		
Na^+	135	mmol/L	
K^+	4.5	mmol/L	
Cl^-	114	mmol/L	
Urea	10	mmol/L	
Creatinine	98	µmol/L	
Lactate	1.3mmol/L		

QUESTION 3.8

A 58 year old male with a history of alcoholism presents with severe central abdominal pain.

His vital signs are:

HR	102	/min
BP	136/98 mmHg	
RR	25	/min
Sats	100%	RA
T	37.4	°C

An arterial blood gas is taken.

FiO_2	0.21		
pH	7.23		
pO_2	101	mmHg	(13.5 kPa)
pCO_2	33	mmHg	(4.4 kPa)
HCO_3^-	18	mmol/L	
BE	-6		
Na^+	142	mmol/L	
K^+	5.1	mmol/L	
Cl^-	106	mmol/L	
Urea	5.2	mmol/L	
Creatinine	76	µmol/L	
Lactate	2.9	mmol/L	

QUESTION 3.9

A 50 year old woman presents after a fire on her boat with a decreased level of consciousness.

Her vital signs are:

HR	122	/min
BP	131/88 mmHg	
RR	32	/min
Sats	100%	60% O_2
T	37.7	°C

An arterial blood gas is taken.

FiO_2	0.6		
pH	7.2		
pO_2	410	mmHg	(54.6 kPa)
pCO_2	26	mmHg	(3.5 kPa)
HCO_3^-	12	mmol/L	
BE	-10		
Na^+	144	mmol/L	
K^+	5.8	mmol/L	
Cl^-	105	mmol/L	
Urea	3.2	mmol/L	
Creatinine	67	µmol/L	
Lactate	3.8	mmol/L	
HbCO	26%		

QUESTION 3.10

A 49 year old woman presents to your department complaining of weight gain and lethargy over the prior month. She is takes no medication.

Her vital signs are:

HR	80	/min
BP	165/90	mmHg
RR	12	/min
Sats	98%	RA
T	37.1	oC

An arterial blood gas is taken.

FiO_2	0.21		
pH	7.55		
PO_2	108	mmHg	(14.4kPa)
PCO_2	49	mmHg	(6.5 kPa)
HCO_3^-	35	mmol/L	
BE	+11		
O2 Sats	98%		
Na^+	153	mmol/L	
K^+	2.1	mmol/L	
Cl^-	129	mmol/L	
Glucose	12.6	mmol/L	

EMQ 3 ANSWERS

QUESTION 3.1

1. **Acid base disturbance**
   Respiratory acidosis and compensatory metabolic alkalosis (expect HCO_3^- 28mmol/L acutely or 40mmol/L chronically)
2. **Anion Gap (AG) and Delta Ratio**
   AG not applicable (alkalosis)
   DR not applicable (acidosis)
3. **A-a gradient in mmHg (kPa)**
   -1.5mmHg (1.07 kPa)
4. **Other relevant calculations**
   Nil applicable
5. **Diagnosis.**
   Death Adder envenomation.

Comment: *Uniquely among the venomous Australian snakes, Death Adders cause isolated respiratory paralysis without rhabdomyolysis or coagulopathy.*

QUESTION 3.2

1. **Acid base disturbance**
   Metabolic acidosis and compensatory respiratory alkalosis.
2. **Anion Gap (AG) and Delta Ratio**
   AG 18
   DR 0.54
3. **A-a gradient in mmHg (kPa)**
   9.25mmHg (2.2 kPa)
4. **Other relevant calculations**
   Urea:creatinine ratio 52
5. **Diagnosis.**
   Drug induced renal failure.

Comment: *This patient has acute intrinsic renal failure, indicated by an isolated rise in creatinine above urea. The combination of NSAIDs, loop diuretics and ACE inhibitors has been associated with renal failure in the literature, and is responsible here for a mixed metabolic acidosis.*

QUESTION 3.3

1. **Acid base disturbance**

   Metabolic acidosis and compensatory respiratory alkalosis (expected CO_2 12mmHg).
2. **Anion Gap (AG) and Delta Ratio**

   AG 33

   DR 1.0
3. **A-a gradient in mmHg (kPa)**

   23mmHg (3.1 kPa)
4. **Other relevant calculations**

   Nil applicable.
5. **Diagnosis.**

   Diabetic ketoacidosis.

Comment: *The combination of significant hyperglycaemia and raised anion gap acidosis indicates a diagnosis of new (and very severe) DKA.*

QUESTION 3.4

1. **Acid base disturbance**

   Metabolic acidosis and compensatory respiratory alkalosis (expect CO_2 29mmHg).
2. **Anion Gap (AG) and Delta Ratio**

   AG 17

   DR 0.5
3. **A-a gradient in mmHg (kPa)**

   8.75mmHg (2.1 kPa)
4. **Other relevant calculations**

   Urea:creatinine ratio 108
5. **Diagnosis.**

   Hyperlactataemia due to perforated duodenal ulcer.

Comment: *This rather ill patient has a mixed metabolic acidosis due to a combination of hyperlactataemia and renal failure, most likely because of a perforated duodenal ulcer as suggested by the stem.*

QUESTION 3.5

1. **Acid base disturbance**

Combined metabolic and respiratory acidosis.

2. **Anion Gap (AG) and Delta Ratio**

   AG 8

   DR not applicable (AG <12)

3. **A-a gradient in mmHg (kPa)**

   41.3mmHg (6.98 kPa)

4. **Other relevant calculations**

   Nil applicable.

5. **Diagnosis.**

   Acute adrenal insufficiency.

Comment: *The combination of non anion gap metabolic acidosis and hyponatraemia with hyperkalaemia suggests acute adrenal insufficiency. The seizure is likely secondary to the critically low sodium level.*

QUESTION 3.6

1. **Acid base disturbance**

   Metabolic acidosis.

2. **Anion Gap (AG) and Delta Ratio**

   AG 15

   DR 0.6

3. **A-a gradient in mmHg (kPa)**

   104mmHg (13.8 kPa)

4. **Other relevant calculations**

   Urea:creatinine ratio 113

5. **Diagnosis.**

   Cardiogenic shock.

Comment: *This patient has cardiogenic shock complicated by a type A lactic acidosis (tissue hypoperfusion), acute renal failure with an associated element of NAGMA and resultant left ventricular failure causing pulmonary oedema and a V/Q mismatch.*

QUESTION 3.7

1. **Acid base disturbance**

   Metabolic acidosis and compensatory respiratory acidosis (expect CO_2 29mmHg).

2. **Anion Gap (AG) and Delta Ratio**

AG 7
DR not applicable (AG <12)

3. **A-a gradient in mmHg (kPa)**
   11.75mmHg (2.5 kPa)
4. **Other relevant calculations**
   Urea:creatinine ratio 10.
5. **Diagnosis.**
   Acetazolamide toxicity.

Comment:*Carbonic anhydrase inhibitors are associated with a non anion gap metabolic acidosis.*

QUESTION 3.8

1. **Acid base disturbance**
   Metabolic acidosis and compensatory respiratory alkalosis (expect CO_2 35mmHg).
2. **Anion Gap (AG) and Delta Ratio**
   AG 18
   DR 1.0
3. **A-a gradient in mmHg (kPa)**
   7.7mmHg (2 kPa)
4. **Other relevant calculations**
   Nil applicable.
5. **Diagnosis.**
   Acute pancreatitis.

Comment: *Although not strictly speaking a cause of raised anion gap metabolic acidosis, alcoholic pancreatitis may be associated with an alcoholic or starvation ketoacidosis, or a lactic acidosis due to associated hypo-perfusion.*

QUESTION 3.9

1. **Acid base disturbance**
   Metabolic acidosis and compensatory respiratory alkalosis (expect CO_2 26mmHg).
2. **Anion Gap (AG) and Delta Ratio**
   AG 27
   DR 1.25

3. **A-a gradient in mmHg (kPa)**
   7.5 mmHg (1 kPa)
4. **Other relevant calculations**
   Nil applicable
5. **Diagnosis.**
   Carbon monoxide toxicity.

Comment: *The history of fire, raised HbCO and hyperoxic tissue hypoxia manifesting as a raised lactate denote acute carbon monoxide toxicity.*

QUESTION 3.10

1. **Acid base disturbance**
   Metabolic alkalosis and compensatory respiratory acidosis (expect CO_2 48mmHg).
2. **Anion Gap (AG) and Delta Ratio**
   AG not applicable (alkalosis)
   DR not applicable (alkalosis)
3. **A-a gradient in mmHg (kPa)**
   0mmHg (0 kPa)
4. **Other relevant calculations**
   Nil applicable.
5. **Diagnosis.**
   Cushing's syndrome.

Comment: *The history of weight gain associated with significant hypernatraemia, hypokalaemia and metabolic alkalosis suggest a diagnosis of Cushing's syndrome.*

THE APPENDICES

"Success is not final, failure is not fatal: it is the courage to continue that counts"

Winston Churchill

Appendix 1: Anion Gap and Delta Ratio

A note on Anion Gap: what are the correct numbers?[59]

Candidates often express a degree of confusion about what constitutes the "normal" value of anion gap, and whether it should be calculated using potassium or not.

The authors' personal opinions are that adding complexity to an already stressful situation (ie the fellowship exam) is unnecessary, and thus any calculations should be as simple as possible. It is surprising under time pressure how difficult adding 4 and 17 can be!

Therefore this book uses an anion gap of 12, based on a calculation without potassium:

$$\textbf{ANION GAP} = [Na+] - ([Cl^-] + [HCO_3-])$$

Reference ranges:

> 12: indicates a raised anion gap metabolic acidosis (RAGMA). A delta ratio should be calculated to evaluate the concurrence of either a NAGMA or a metabolic alkalosis

< or equal to 12: indicates a NAGMA. A delta ratio is not performed

It is worth noting however that a NAGMA can present with a mildly raised anion gap (above 12). This is because there is not a discrete anion gap cut off for "normal" or "raised" values. Most papers specify an anion gap without K^+ as having a normal value of 12 +/- 4. Thus even in the event of an anion gap greater than 12, the possibility of a NAGMA should be considered, and a delta ratio calculation performed to evaluate for the possibility.

For those with more interest in the subject a good place to start is with reading the reference below.

---

59 Lolekha PH, Vanavanan S and Lolekha S. (2001) Update on value of the anion gap in clinical diagnosis and laboratory evaluation. *Clin Chim Acta* 307 (1-2): 33 – 36

The Delta Ratio[60]

Delta ratio is defined as (change in AG)/(change in HCO_3^-). It is calculated by:

$$\frac{AG - 12}{24 - [HCO_3^-]}$$

A delta ratio is interpreted as follows:

< 0.4 (large drop in HCO_3^- without change in AG) = NAGMA

0.4 – 0.8 (intermittent drop in AG compared to HCO_3^-) = NAGMA + RAGMA

1.0 (equal drop in HCO_3^- and AG) = RAGMA

2.0+ (lower drop HCO_3^- in than expected for AG) = there is a previously existing or concurrent metabolic alkalosis occurring. Mathematically this ratio occurs *because the resting HCO_3^- for the patient is greater than 24mmol/L*

---

60 Kim HY, Han JS, Jeon US, Joo KW, Earm JH, Ahn C et al. (2001). Clinical significance of the fractional excretion of anions in metabolic acidosis. *Clin Nephrol* 2001 55(6): 448-52

Appendix 2: Assessing Compensation

The reference[61] given is not the original paper on correcting acid base balances, but provides a very good overview of acid-base balance in general, and correction rules in particular. The correction calculations follow.

For primary metabolic acidosis:

Expected CO_2 in mmHg = 8 + 1.5 x $[HCO_3^-]$

For primary metabolic alkalosis:

Expected CO_2 in mmHg = 21 + 0.7 x $[HCO_3^-]$

For primary respiratory acidosis:

$[HCO_3^-]$ increases by 1mmol/L per 10mmHg CO_2 above 40mmHg

$[HCO_3^-]$ increases by 4mmol/L per 10mmHg CO_2 above 40mmHg

For primary respiratory alkalosis:

$[HCO_3^-]$ decreases by 2mmol/L per 10mmHg CO_2 below 40mmHg

$[HCO_3^-]$ decreases by 5mmol/L per 10mmHg CO_2 below 40mmHg

61 Sood P, Gunchan P and Sandeep P (2010). Interpretation of arterial blood gas. *Indian J Crit Care Med* 14(2): 57 - 64

Appendix 3: Notes on Sundry Calculations

A-a Gradient[62]

The equation to calculate an A-a gradient in mmHg is:

$$[(760\text{-vapour pressure}) \times FiO_2 - 1.25 \times PaCO_2) - PaO_2$$

One of the hardest things in the exam is trying to calculate the P_AO_2 ([760-vapour pressure] x FiO_2) for an FiO_2 that's not room air.

This is the most obvious instance in the examination where approximation is acceptable:

- If FiO_2 = 21% (room air) then the first number in the equation (760-VP x FiO_2) is 150mmHg.
- By dead reckoning, FiO_2 40% then the first number is doubled: 300mmHg
- Similarly on 28% O_2 (somewhere in the ballpark of 1.3 x 21…) 200mmHg (1.0 x 150mmHg) can be used

A standard comment in the event of an elevated A-a gradient is:

"A-a gradient elevated. ∴ V/Q mismatch:

- *APO*
- *ARDS*
- *PE*
- *LRTI*
- *Other respiratory membrane disease*

There is some discussion of this particularly as it pertains to pneumonia in the associated reference.

For those using the calculations in kPa it is important to realise that atmospheric pressure (after water vapour is removed) at sea level is

---

62 Moammar MQ, Azam HM, Blamoun AI, Rashid AO, Ismail M, Khan MA et al. (2008). Alveolar-arterial oxygen gradient, pneumonia severity index and outcomes in patients hospitalized with community acquired pneumonia. *Clin Exp Pharmacol Physiol* 35(9): 1032-7

101kPa. This means that the first number in the A-a gradient calculation (the FiO_2) is equal to the percentage of administered oxygen. There is no easily applied formal corrective formula for age when kPa are used to calculate A-a gradient, and normal values cited in the literature vary. As a rule of thumb young people should have an A-a gradient between 2.5 – 3.0 kPa, while older people (60+) should have an A-a gradient <4.0 kPa[63].

Electrolytes

Sodium[64]

$$\text{Corrected } Na^+ = Na^+_m + (\text{Glucose} - 5)/3.$$

This is very important for DKA cases. The experimental numbers for absolute sodium vary but the equation above is a useful approximation for the exam.

Potassium[65]

Potassium homeostasis is complex, and varies with the type and mechanism of acidaemia or alkalaemia. Practically, for exam purposes for each pH fall below 7.4, K^+ should rise by 0.5mmol above 5.0mmol/L. Therefore an appropriate comment would be along the lines of:

> *K^+ 4.0mmol/L = normal.*
> *Expect K^+ for pH 7.2 = 5.0 + 2 x 0.5 = 6.0mmol/L.*
> *.: pt relatively hypokalaemic. Watch/replace K^+ as pH corrected.*

Renal indices[66]

---

63 Williams AJ. Assessing and interpreting arterial blood gases and acid-base balance. *BMJ* 1998; 317(7167): 1213 – 1216.3

64 Hillier TA, Abbott RD and Barrett EJ. (1999) Hyponatraemia: evaluating the correction factor for hyperglycaemia. *Am J Med* 106(4): 399 – 403.

65 Rastegar A. Clinical Methods: the History, Physical and Laboratory Examinations. 3rd Ed. Chapter 195 Boston, *Butterworths*; 1990

66 Feinfeld DA, Bargouthi H, Niaz Q, Carvounis CP. (2002) Massive and disproportionate elevation of blood urea nitrogen in acute azotaemia. *Int urol nephrol* 34(1) 143:145

When assessing urea to creatinine ratio the examination answer is almost always ~100 and therefore suggests pre-renal failure. Again this is a gross simplification, but unless the number is very low (<50 indicating intrinsic renal failure) it is a useful mechanism for the exam.

Osmolality[67]

The only reason to give candidates a measured osmolality in the question stem is to enable calculation of an osmolar gap, which is a two step process:

$$\text{Calculated osmolality} = 2 \times Na^{+} + \text{urea} + \text{glucose}$$

$$\text{osmolar gap} = OSM_{m} - OSM_{c}.$$

<u>If there is a measured osmolality in the stem you would be foolish not to perform these calculations.</u>

67 Hoffman RS, Smilkstein MJ, Howland MA and Goldfrank LR. (1993) Osmol gaps revisited: normal values and limitations. *Clin Toxicol,* 31: 81-93.

Appendix 4: ACEM Terminology

"It is always important to read a question carefully, and to understand these terms in the context of that question. The Fellowship Examination Committee and the examiners are instructed to be rigorous in the use of these terms. Candidates are advised to do similarly."[68]

Assessment: History taking, physical examination and investigations.

Describe: State the characteristics or appearance of the subject, including relevant negatives.

Discuss: Examine the pros and cons of each of the alternatives asked for on a subject.

Disposition: Where the patient is sent following care in the emergency department, including follow - up if discharged.

Interpret: State a conclusion or conclusions which includes a differential diagnosis, but excludes management.

Investigations: Specific tests undertaken to make a diagnosis or monitor the patient's condition.

List: A numerical ordering of related items.

Management: Those aspects of care of the patient encompassing treatment, supportive care and disposition.

Outline: A brief description of the subject.

Protocol: A set of instructions on how to deal with a particular situation.

Treatment: Measures undertaken to cure or stabilize the patient's condition

---

68 Australasian College for Emergency Medicine. Examination Handbook v02. Published online and retrieved 18 November 2013 from: http://www.acem.org.au/media/publications/FEH02_v02_Fellowship_Exam_Structure__Mar-12_.pdf

Appendix 5: Luke Lawton's Lists of Causes of Acid-base Disturbances

The following lists are taken from Luke's study notes when preparing for the ACEM fellowship exam. They are illustrative of the type of list for causes of acid-base disorders that candidates should assemble in their minds prior to the exam. In no way are the lists definitive in content or scope and are not specific to any particular reference. The information is essentially an amalgamation of multiple sources compiled during study, arranged in an order pleasing to the author.

Causes of RAGMA

1. Lactic Acid

   A: cyanide toxicity, arterial occlusion (mesenteric ischaemia), hypovolaemia, profound anaemia

   B_1: liver failure (paracetamol poisoning), sepsis

   B_2: most drugs (methanol, ethylene glycol, paraldehyde, paraquat, iron, isoniazid, metformin)

   B_3: inborn errors of metabolism

2. Ketoacids

   Diabetic ketoacidosis
   Starvation/alcoholic ketoacidosis

3. Salicylates

4. Uraemic renal failure

Causes of NAGMA

1. HCO_3^- loss (most common)
    Excessive diarrhoea
    Renal tubular acidosis
    Fistulas (pancreaticoduodenal, uretoenteric)

2. Excessive 0.9% NaCl administration

3. Endocrinopathies
    Mineralocorticoid or glucocorticoid deficiency
    Adrenal crisis

4. Drugs
    Carbonic anhydrase inhibitors (acetazolamide)
    Spironolactone

Causes of metabolic alkalosis

1. HCl loss (most common)
    Vomiting

2. Drug induced
    Diuretics (esp frusemide)
    Laxative abuse
    Milk-alkali syndrome
    NaHCO3 therapy

3. Endocrinopathies
    Mineralocorticoid or glucocorticoid excess
    Bartter's syndrome

Causes of respiratory alkalosis

1. Central stimulation of respiratory drive
   - Head injury/ICH
   - Anxiety/pain
   - Salicylate intoxication
   - Sympathomimmetic intoxication (MDMA etc)

2. Profound hypoxia causing peripheral respiratory stimulation
   - PE, pneumonia, pulmonary oedema, acute asthma, ARDS

Causes of respiratory acidosis

1. Acute on chronic exacerbation of COAD

2. Airway disorders
   - Acute asthma
   - Airway obstruction

3. Depression of central respiratory drive
   - Drugs (opiates, sedatives)
   - ICH, CNS injury

4. Lung insults
   - Trauma (pulmonary contusion, pneumothorax, haemothorax, flail segment)
   - Lung membrane diseases (pulmonary oedema, lower respiratory tract infection, ARDS, aspiration)

5. Inadequate respiratory effort
   - Toxins (organophosphates, elapid envenomation)
   - Myopathies, Guillain-Barre syndrome

Notes.

About the Authors

Associate Professor Luke Lawton holds degrees in biochemistry, medicine, surgery and public health, and is a Fellow of the Australasian College for Emergency Medicine. He works as an emergency physician at Townsville University Hospital in North Queensland and teaches at James Cook University's College of Medicine and Dentistry. His educational interests include undergraduate medical teaching and the preparation of ACEM Fellowship candidates through his local health service. He is a member of the EMCORE faculty and Chair of the Editorial Committee for the 12th Edition of the *Primary Clinical Care Manual.* Clinically, his focus is intelligent medicine. and doing the right thing for his patients.

In addition to medical writing, he is the author of the historical espionage novel *Four Nights in France.*

Dr Corinne Ryan is a Fellow of the Royal Australian College of Physicians and specializes in medical oncology. She has a biochemistry degree from Queensland University of Technology and studied medicine at James Cook University where she is now an adjunct senior lecturer with the College of Medicine and Dentistry. She is enthusiastic about clinical teaching of undergraduates and doctors in training, and has provided specialist medical comment on many of the topics in this book.

www.ingramcontent.com/pod-product-compliance
Lightning Source LLC
LaVergne TN
LVHW070909210926
848482LV00017B/1030

* 9 7 8 0 9 9 2 4 2 4 5 5 8 *